Beginning Yoga

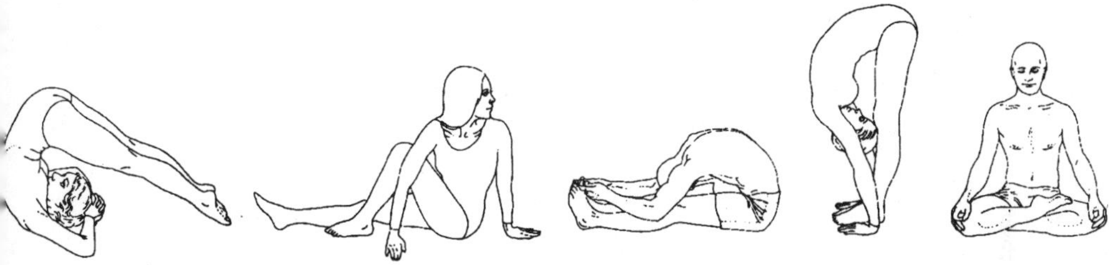

by Vijayendra Pratap, Ph. D., D. Y. P.

SKY Foundation
Philadelphia, Pennsylvania, U. S. A.

TUTTLE PUBLISHING
Boston • Rutland, Vermont • Tokyo

First published in 1960 by Tuttle Publishing, an imprint of Periplus Editions (HK) Ltd., with editorial offices at 153 Milk Street, Boston, Massachusetts, 02109.

Library of Congress Cataloging-in-Publication Data

LCC Card No. 60-6926
ISBN 0-8048-2104-6

Distributed by:

North America
Tuttle Publishing
Distribution Center
Airport Industrial Park
364 Innovation Drive
North Clarendon, VT 05759-9436
Tel: (802) 773-8930
Fax: (802) 773-6993

Japan
Tuttle Publishing
RK Building, 2nd Floor
2-13-10 Shimo-Meguro
Meguro-Ku
Tokyo 153 0064
Tel: (03) 5437-0171
Fax: (03) 5437-0755

Asia Pacific
Berkeley Books Pte Ltd
130 Joo Seng Road
#06-01/03 Olivine Building
Singapore 368357
Tel: (65) 6280-1330
Fax: (65) 6280-6290

08 07 06 05 04 03 02 15 14 13 12 11 10

Printed in the United States of America

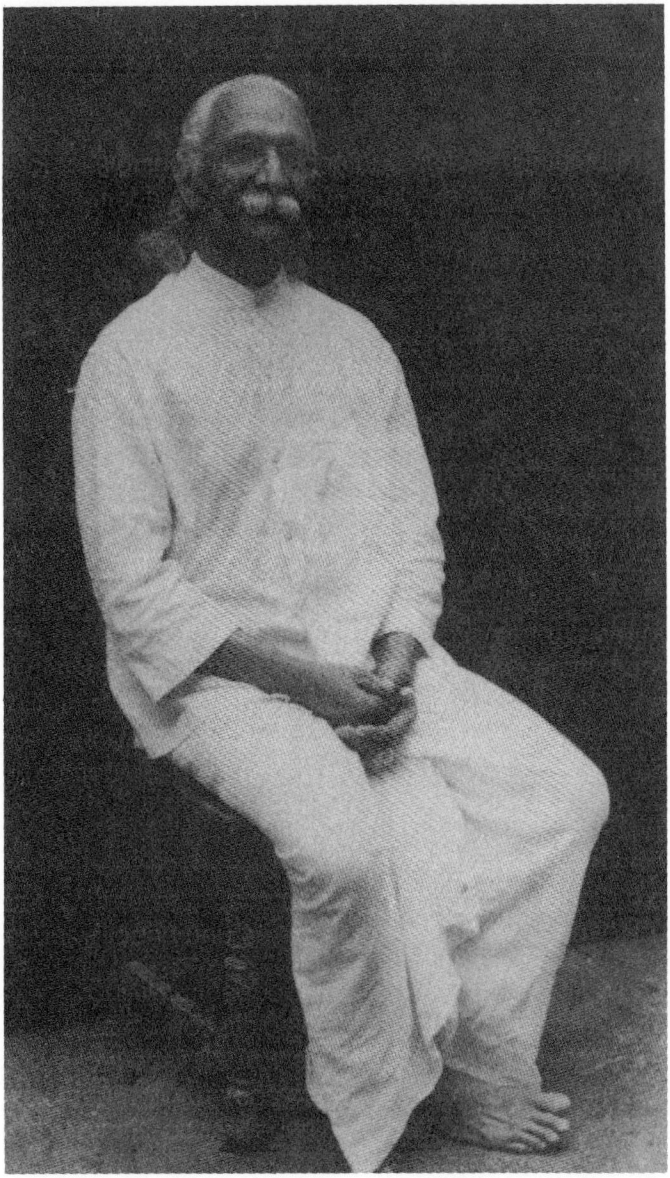

My Teacher

Swâmî Kuvalayânandaji (1883-1966)
Scientifically-minded Yogi
Founder of the Kaivalyadhâma Institutions
and inspiration for SKY Foundation

Photograph courtesy of Kaivalyadhâma, Lonavla, INDIA

Dedicated
to
My Revered Teacher
and Teachers

KAIVALYADHAMA

Shriman Madhava Yoga Mandir Samiti

An Institute for Scientific and Philosophico – Literary Research, Training & Treatment in Yoga

ॐ

सोऽहम् ।

Phone : 339

Please address your reply to:

The Chairman,
KAIVALYADHAMA
LONAVLA 410 403 (India)

Ref. No. K/

Date : ....

ॐ

स्वस्तिरस्तु · श्रीरस्तु

Digambar

OM

"Let wellness and prosperity be bestowed upon you."

Swami Digambarji

Abbreviations

Â.	*Âsanas*
D.U.	*Daršanopaniṣad*
Gh.S.	*Gheraṇḍa Saṁhitâ*
GÎTÂ	*Šrîmadbhagavadgîtâ*
G.Š.	*Gorakṣa Šatakam*
H.P.	*Haṭha-Pradîpikâ*
M.U.	*Muṇḍaka Upaniṣad*
P.	*Prâṇâyâma*
P.Y.S.	*Patañjali's Yoga Sûtras*
Ṣ.C.N.	*Ṣaṭ-Cakra-Nirûpaṇa*
S.S.P.	*Siddha-Siddhânta-Paddhati*
Š.S.	*Šiva-Saṁhitâ*
T.Š.B.	*Trišikhibrâhmṇopaniṣad*
V.U.	*Varâhopaniṣad*
Y.K.U.	*Yogakuṇḍalinyupaniṣad*
Y.T.	*Yogic Therapy*

SYSTEM OF TRANSLITERATION

(IN ENGLISH ALPHABETICAL ORDER)

LETTERS	PRONUNCIATION	SAṀSKṚTA
a	sun	अ
â	art	आ
ai	aisle	ऐ
au	house	औ
b	bow	ब्
bh	abhor	भ्
c	chariot	च्
ch	charge	छ्
d	then	द्
ḍ	devotion	ड्
dh	this	ध्
ḍh	adhere	ढ्
e	sage	ए
g	God	ग्
gh	ghost	घ्
h	hut	ह्
ḥ	aha	ः
i	sit	इ
î	seat	ई
j	joy	ज्
jh	hedgehog	झ्
jñ	jñâna	ज्ञ्
k	calm	क्
kh	Eckhart	ख्
kṣ	Lakṣmî	क्ष्

LETTERS	PRONUNCIATION	SAṀSKṚTA
l	love	ल्
m	monk	म्
ṁ	momentum	ं
n	nose	न्
ṇ	tender	ण्
ṅ	king	ङ्
ñ	Señor	ञ्
o	home	ओ
p	patience	प्
ph	philosophy	फ्
r	road	र्
ṛ	merrily	ऋ
s	seer	स्
ṣ	shut	ष्
š	sure	श्
t	thin	त्
ṭ	twist	ट्
th	thought	थ्
ṭh	anthill	ठ्
u	pull	उ
û	wool	ऊ
v	value	व्
w	swâmî	व्
y	yoke	य्

Contents

BLESSINGS FROM SWAMI DIGAMBARJI

ACKNOWLEDGMENTS

FIRST BREATH 15

HELPFUL HINTS 18

ŠAVÂSANA (Corpse Pose) 21

BHUJAṄGÂSANA (Cobra Pose) 23

ARDHA-ŠALABHÂSANA (Half-Locust Pose) 26

ŠALABHÂSANA (Locust Pose) 28

DHANURÂSANA (Bow Pose) 30

MAKARÂSANA (Crocodile Pose) 32

ARDHA-HALÂSANA (Half-Plow Pose) First Stage 34

ARDHA-HALÂSANA + (Half-Plow Pose) Second Stage 36

HALÂSANA (Plow Pose) 38

DAṆḌÂSANA (Stick Pose) 41

VAKRÂSANA (Twist Pose) 43

ARDHA-MATSYENDRÂSANA (Half-Matsyendra Pose) 46

PAŠCIMATÂNÂSANA (Posterior Stretch Pose) 49

STAMBHÂSANA (Pillar Pose) 52

CAKRÂSANA (Side-Bending Pose) 54

VṚKṢÂSANA (Tree Pose) 57

SAṄKAṬÂSANA (Difficult Pose) 60

PÂDAHASTÂSANA (Hand-to-Foot Pose) 63

VAJRÂSANA (Pelvic Pose) 65

SUKHÂSANA (Easy Pose) 68

VÎRÂSANA (Hero Pose) 71

SVASTIKÂSANA (Auspicious Pose) 74

PADMÂSANA (Lotus Pose) 76

YOGA MUDRÂ (Symbol of Yoga) 79

BRAHMA MUDRÂ (Symbol of Brahmâ) 82

UJJÂYÎ (Breathing with Sound) First Stage 85

UJJÂYÎ + (Breathing with Sound) Second Stage 88

PRACTICE PLANS 91

GLOSSARY 109

REFERENCES 119

Acknowledgments

Preparation of this manuscript began in 1972. In 1976, Swâmî Digambarji, Director of Research, Kaivalyadhâma, S. M. Y. M. Samiti, reviewed it and gave his blessings. I am greatly indebted to him for his teaching and advice; and appreciative of the support I've received from Šrî O. P. Tiwari and my Ašramite brothers.

This project also owes a great deal to the students and sustaining members of the SKY Foundation who have supported my work over the years. Special thanks to those who posed for the drawings used in this guide: Marc Goldberg, Barbara Levitt, Gershon Levitt, Belinda Owens, Candace Smith, and Katherine Da Silva Jain. Susan Richards, Linda Gross, and Anne Craig provided assistance in the early stages of this book, and for this I am grateful.

In preparing this book finally for publishing, I depended on the hard work, devotion, and persistence of Barbara Levitt who was responsible for its layout, typesetting, and mechanical composition. She was aided in her computer work by Richard Friedman and B. J. Levitt, and shared copyediting responsibilities with Judy Friedman and Gershon Levitt.

Joan Krejcar was enthusiastic in her work on the illustrations.

A very special thanks to Candace Smith of the Garland of Letters Bookstore, to Margaret Smith James, and to my Mother for their advice and encouragement throughout.

I also express my appreciation to Margo Evans and Charles Blanken of Science Press for their technical assistance.

I feel confident that this book will be helpful to teachers and students alike. I would be happy to have their comments and suggestions for future projects.

I never thought, when I began, that such a small book would require so much effort from so many. May God bless them all.

कर्मण्येवाधिकारस्ते मा फलेषु कदाचन ।

Work is only thy duty.
Result is not thy concern.

Gîtâ II, 47

शरीरमाद्यं खलु धर्मसाधनम् ।

Surely health is the primary requisite of spiritual life.

Kâlîdâsa (*Kumârasambhava* V. 33)

The First Breath

This manual of easy poses is designed to help both teachers and students interested in beginning Yoga to learn postures and some preliminary breathing practices.

There are currently hundreds of books that meet the needs of many students and teachers of Yoga. This differs in that it uses modern terminology to bring sincere students closer to the classical tradition. In the process, emphasis is laid not only on the physical aspect of each pose, but also on the underlying subtleties of that pose.

The plan of this work is as follows:

Technique

This section includes step-by-step instructions for the pose and is accompanied by the appropriate illustrations.

Suggestions

This includes those important learning points which are often overlooked, sometimes for the sake of external appearances, at the cost of the psycho-physiological effects of the pose.

Results

This section suggests benefits that may be derived from the pose, either described in traditional texts or discovered as a result of modern scientific research in the field of Yogic therapy.

Discussion and References

The meaning of the pose, whether classical or modern, is given and an explanation of its name is offered. Sources are cited of those poses which are ancient.

A pose is an attitude which has two aspects: physical and mental. The physical aspect may be related to something in nature, such as an animal, plant, or an object. The mental aspect of a pose may be symbolic, subtle, or involve mythological concepts, an understanding of which is very useful for healthy living.

According to the Haṭha Yoga tradition, the number of Âsanas range from 2 to 84, and up to 8,400,000 (84 Lacs) "...as many as there are species of animals" (*G.Š.* 5, 6 & 7; *Š.S.* III, 84; and *Gh.S.* II, 1 & 2).

While some postures take their inspiration from the natural world, such as Lotus, Cobra, Locust and Tree Poses – others were originated to stimulate certain centers of the body and afterwards their resemblances were noted (this is probably the case in the Plow and Bow Poses).

It is helpful, as you practice each pose, to be aware of its background and the relationship to these underlying meanings. The body is, after all, only the medium through which you approach higher states. Yoga is a fine art based on sound scientific principles. It is an integrated way of life.

Yoga teaches that you are the master of your own destiny. You, yourself, hold the key to a productive life of contentment and inner peace.

This key is self-discipline.

Too often, today, the word "discipline" brings a negative reaction. We think of painful austerity and deprivation. But this is not the discipline of Yoga.

Properly followed – that is, with respect and for a long period of time – Yogic training will beautify your life. As you bring yourself into a state of balance and harmony, a new consciousness will dawn upon you. You will find a disciplined life to be one filled with its own joys and rewards.

Posture is one important Yogic tool. Adjusting your attitude through the medium of your body leads to emotional stability, health, and suppleness.

Regarding the order of postures, there is no authoritative agreement. No doubt, there is a systematic hierarchy in Yoga for posture, Prâṇâyâma, Mudrâ, and meditative practices. Maharṣi Patañjali, in his *Yoga Sûtras*, gives an eightfold path that includes: Yama, Niyama, Âsana, Prâṇâyâma, Pratyâhâra, Dhâraṇâ, Dhyâna, and Samâdhi.

If there is a hierarchy, however, among the postures themselves, a good deal of research must yet be done to accurately determine it.

In this book, I will follow closely the teachings of Swâmî Kuvalayânandaji, who devoted much of his life to the systematic, scientific study of classical Yoga.

This *Teacher's Guide for Beginning Yoga* provides a step-by-step approach for those who wish to make a beginning.

If you follow the practices outlined in this book for some time with enthusiasm and respect, you will reach a new level of well-being.

What is most important at first, however, is to begin.

Best wishes!

Helpful Hints

1. Yogic practices bring appreciable results if done continuously, for a long period, and with respect. However, whatever is done in a proper way, will not be a waste. Of course, regular practice has a more profound effect.

2. Practices with a light stomach lead to feelings of well-being. Therefore, avoid heavy meals for about three hours before practice, and also snacks for about an hour. Moderate food, which is appropriate and conducive to the healthy way of living, is advocated. A pleasant attitude while eating food is as important as the food itself.

3. Choose a place for practice that is quiet and well ventilated, free from draft and din. Burn some mild incense. Have some inspiring photographs, pictures, or concepts, which may be helpful and bring to your consciousness again and again what you want to accomplish. These arrangements will create an atmosphere that will be helpful to Yogic practice.

4. Have a nice seat for your practices. The traditional arrangement of the seat for the spiritual aspirant is Kuša grass, i.e., a grass mat, and above that a tiger, lion, or deer skin covered by a piece of cloth. If you do not feel comfortable with the idea of skin, use a woolen blanket and cover with a washable, clean cloth.

5. Choose a time for practice. You can decide, after some days of practices, which time is best for you. This will condition you for practices and free you from fighting the idea of whether or not to do it.

6. Take a whole bath or shower before you do your practices, or at least wash your face, hands, and feet. You will feel fresh with a feeling of purity. This feeling can be brought about in several ways: water, Mantra, exposure to sun, air, etc.

7. Wear loose or stretchable clothing while you practice so that blood flow, breathing, and movement will be easy and unrestricted.
8. Approach Yoga with the spirit of a sportsman, having an attitude that will lead to success and beyond. It is a question of values when you choose something to do.
9. Do not be a perfectionist. Individuals differ in their physical and mental abilities, so avoid comparing yourself with others. This is one of the secrets of happy living.
10. With regard to the practices, do not strain, and whenever you feel the need for rest during practice, relax. The Corpse and Crocodile Poses are good for relaxation.
11. The process, the way you do it, is more important than the final position. It will help you develop the Yogic attitude toward what you do in a calm, secure, contented way.
12. Follow the order of poses in such a way that the poses complement each other, and include all the possible movements of the spine. If you cannot do some practices, work on them slowly, gradually, and patiently. It is your own body – it needs training and not straining.
13. Pairing physically strenuous exercises with Yogic practices at the same time is not desirable. It is always better to have one in the morning and the other in the evening. As an alternative, the two could be practiced with a break of at least 15-20 minutes between them.
14. Let breathing take care of itself while you are doing Âsanas, or "postures." When you feel like exhaling, exhale, and when you feel like inhaling, inhale; i.e., breathing should be allowed to proceed as normally as possible. There are, however, other practices where breathing and postures are combined – these need caution.

15. Start and end your practices with an attitude of devotion, with eyes closed, by chanting "Om" three times or so. Or just sit quietly with eyes closed and be aware of your breath.
16. If you fail to do your practices, do not be disheartened. Try again. Persistence is the key to great achievements in life.
17. Of course, there is no substitute for personal help and instruction from a competent teacher. If you really want and need guidance, you will find it.
18. Start today!

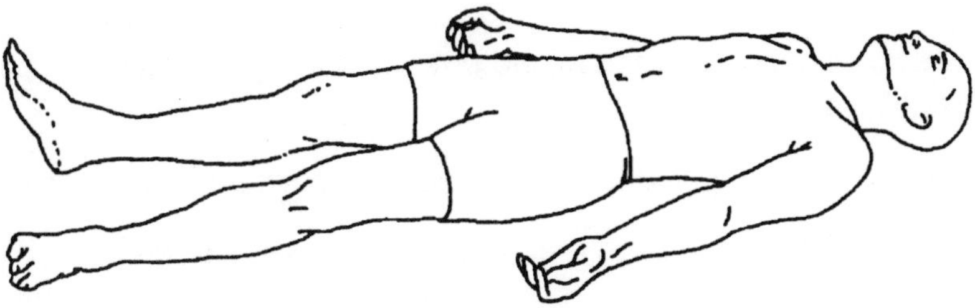

I

ŠAVÂSANA

Corpse Pose

Technique

Lie supine, with feet comfortably apart and relaxed, hands at a comfortable distance along the sides of the body, with palms up and eyes closed.

Be aware of your breath – incoming and outgoing.

Suggestions

1. Eyes closed, unless you are uncomfortable with eyes closed.
2. Pay attention to the flow of your breath. It is easier for many to feel the flow at the tip of the nostrils.
3. Rest your head wherever it feels comfortable.
4. If you find a tendency to fall asleep during Šavâsana, try bringing your feet closer together.

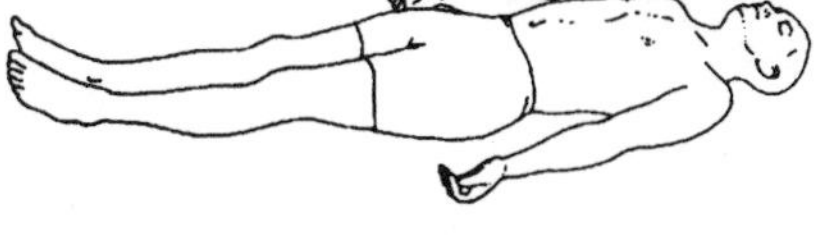

Results

Šavâsana overcomes mental and physical fatigue, and also provides a sense of well-being.

It helps to reduce tensions and enables the development of insight.

The mastering of this pose may help make a person free from the fear of death.

This pose may be prescribed for terminal patients with great advantage.

Discussion and References

Šava means corpse. Âsana means pose. Therefore, Šavâsana means Corpse Pose.

Gh.S. II, 19 describes it as Mṛtâsana. Mṛta means dead. It is, therefore, synonymous with Šavâsana. *H.P.* I, 32 also describes the pose with slight variations.

Corpse Pose is an imitation of the corpse which enables one to learn to die while he or she is still alive. That is, the person having this experience will not be afraid of the idea of death.

Experiencing death may open the gate to a higher state of consciousness.

It will lead a person to a feeling of floating in the sky (Vyomasaṃcâra).

So Šavâsana may lead to Šivâsana, which means the Seat of Lord Šiva.

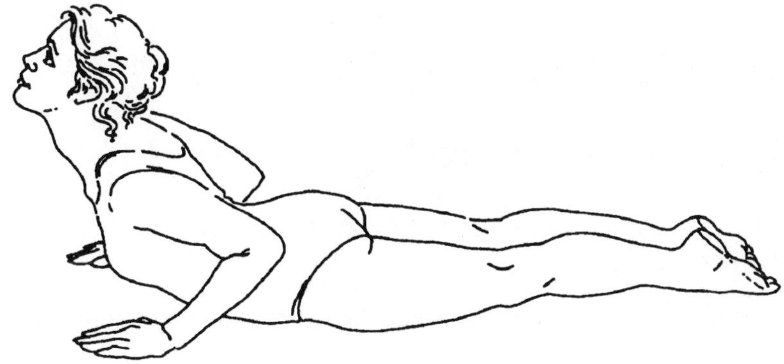

II

BHUJAṄGÂSANA

Cobra Pose

Technique

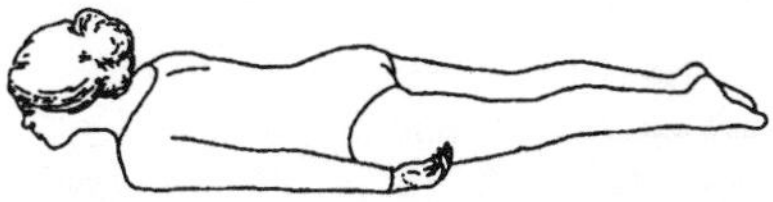

Lie prone and relax.

Place your feet together, forehead on the ground, your arms along the sides of the body.

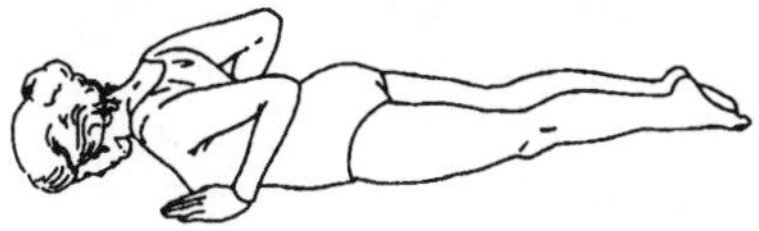

Now place your palms on each side of the chest, thumbs in the line of the nipples, elbows close to the back of the body.

Raise your head slowly and stretch your neck backward. Keep your gaze moving up.

Then raise your chest, gradually curving your spine, vertebra by vertebra. Raise up to the navel only and hold the pose for some time.

Release, and return to your original position, gradually uncurving the back and placing the chest on the ground, then lowering the gaze, and finally placing the arms along the sides of the body.

Repeat three or four times and then relax in Šavâsana (Corpse Pose).

Suggestions

1. Keep your palms close to your body, fingers together, and with elbows bent and stretched toward the spine.
2. Use hands for minimum support, i.e., place minimal weight on the hands.
3. Trunk should be lifted up to the navel only; if you lift beyond, push back down.
4. The whole process of raising the chest and curving the back must be gradual, vertebra by vertebra.
5. Do not raise your feet from the ground when you are raising your head.

Results

The deep muscles of the back become healthy as the spine becomes elastic and blood circulation and tone of the muscles and spinal nerves improve. This pose makes abdominal muscles healthier, removes gases, relieves constipation, and improves digestion.

Discussion and References

Bhujaṅga means cobra, snake, or serpent. Âsana means pose. Therefore, Bhujaṅgâsana means Cobra or Serpent Pose (*Gh.S.* II, 42- 43).

Bhujaṅgâsana is helpful in awakening the Kuṇḍalinî (serpent power or latent energy), which is lying at the root of the spine, known as Mûlâdhâra Cakra.

A snake is also a symbol of energy.

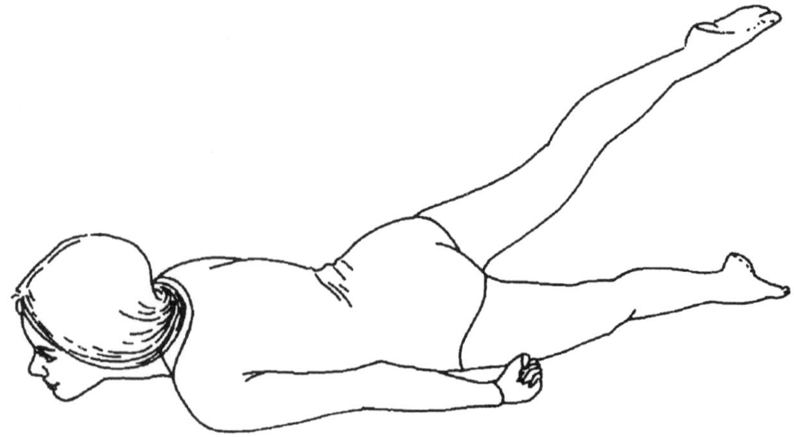

III

ARDHA-ŠALABHÂSANA

Half-Locust Pose

Technique

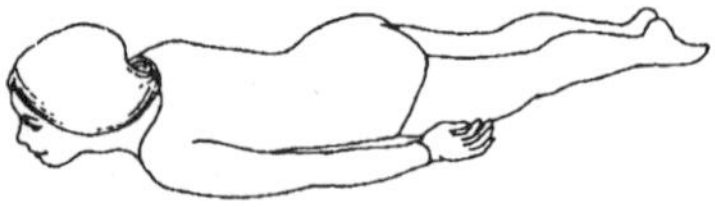

Lie prone, hands along the sides of the body with palms up and chin on the floor.

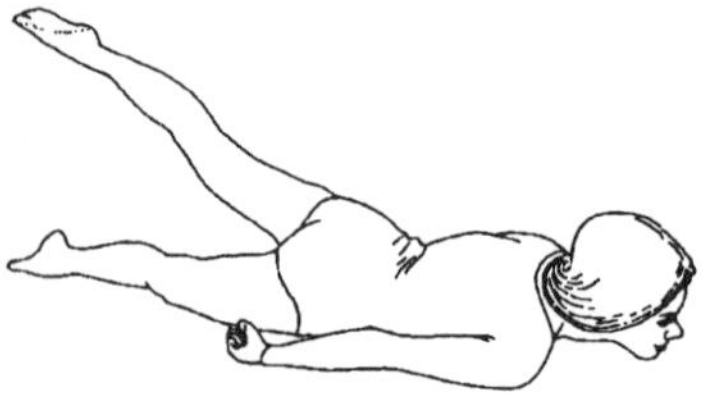

Close your fists and raise your left leg slowly without bending the knees or tilting the body. Hold for some time and bring it back to the original position gradually.

Then raise your right leg in the same manner.

Repeat three or four times.

Relax in either Makarâsana (Crocodile Pose) or Šavâsana (Corpse Pose).

Suggestions

1. Keep the body and the knees straight.
2. Lift the leg gradually.
3. Do not raise your chin when you are lifting your leg.

Results

It is a fine exercise for the abdomen.

Weak persons can also do it.

It is relatively more invigorating for the lower parts of the spine below the navel, while Bhujaṅgâsana deals with the upper part of the spine.

Discussion and References

Ardha means half. Šalabha means locust. Âsana means pose. Therefore, Ardha-Šalabhâsana means Half-Locust Pose.

This is a simpler version of the traditional pose, Locust, as only one leg is raised at a time. See discussion under Šalabhâsana.

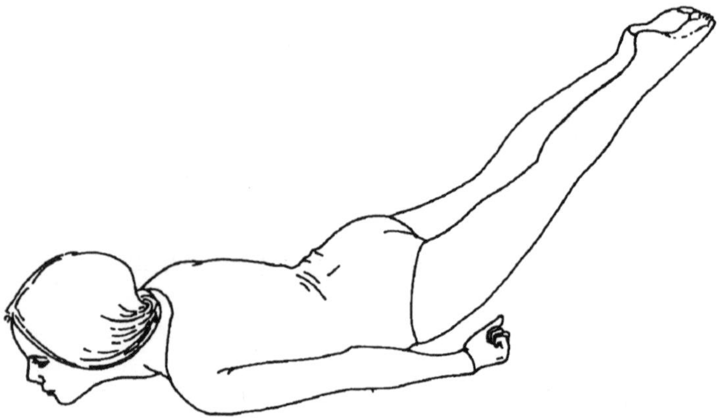

IV

ŠALABHÂSANA

Locust Pose

Technique

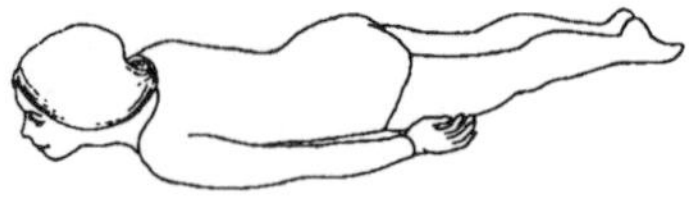

Lie prone, hands along the sides of the body with palms up and chin on the floor.

Close your fists and slowly raise both legs together. Raise as far as you can go, keeping your legs straight.

Hold this pose for some time and then slowly bring back your legs and relax awhile.

Repeat three or four times.

Suggestions

1. Raise the legs together without jerking.
2. Do not bend the legs at the knees.
3. Try to keep your chin and shoulders touching the floor.

4. Return to the original position gradually.
5. Raise the legs from the floor about nine inches and maintain; then go as high as you can, but not beyond the navel.
6. You can also insert your fists under your groin or thighs, keeping your arms straight, to raise the legs more easily.

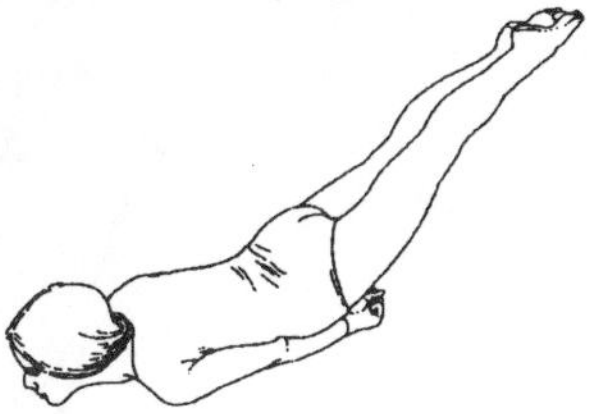

Results

It is a fine exercise for the abdomen. This serves as a complementary pose to the Cobra Pose. It enriches blood circulation in the lower parts of the body and makes the lumbo-sacral nerves healthy.

Discussion and References

Šalabha means locust. Âsana means pose. Therefore, Šalabhâsana means Locust Pose.

This pose resembles the insect, locust. According to *Gheraṇḍa Saṁhitâ*, the palms may be placed near the chest. Šalabha also means grasshopper.

The word Šalabha includes the letters sa, la, and bha. According to the lexicographers, these letters stand for the names of Šiva, Indra, and the planet Šukra (Venus), respectively. "La" is also the secret symbol of the Mûlâdhâra Cakra (anal plexus). It is associated with Pṛthvî Tattva (earth element).

Locusts and grasshoppers have excellent hearing. Their ears are located on the abdomen, at the base of the hindlegs.

It seems that Šalabhâsana is one of those poses which contributes to the arousal of the latent vital force, known as Kuṇḍalinî. Further scientific research work is necessary to fully explain this process.

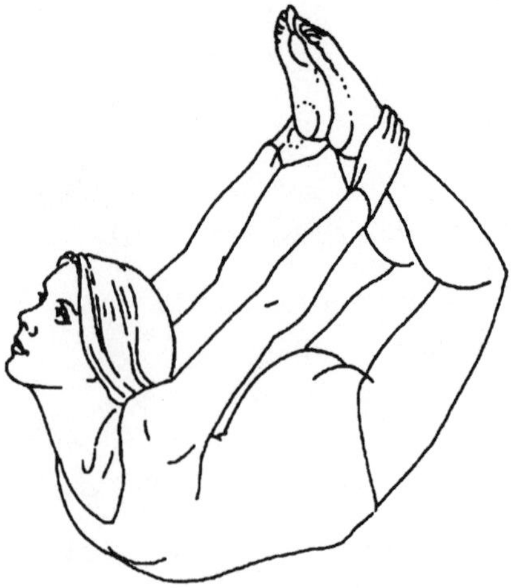

V

DHANURÂSANA

Bow Pose

Technique

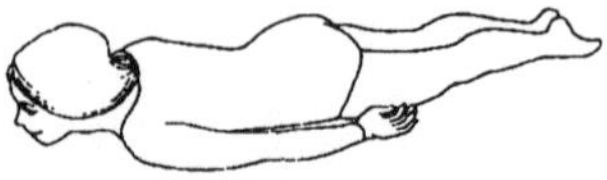

Lie prone, hands along the sides of the body and chin on the floor.

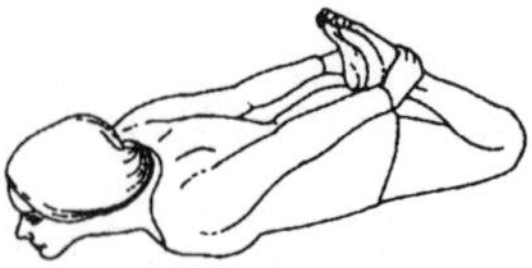

Bend your legs at the knee slowly and catch hold of your ankles.

Raise your knees and trunk together, stretching your neck by bringing your head back as far as possible.

Hold the pose for a few seconds and return to the original position slowly by bringing the chest and knees down, releasing the ankles, and then placing the hands on the floor.

Repeat three or four times.

Suggestions

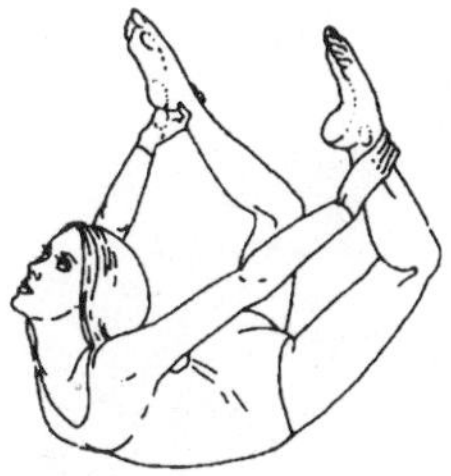

1. Keep the knees apart in the beginning. As you feel comfortable, bring them closer.
2. Try to rest on the navel.
3. Keep the arms straight.
4. Turn your gaze upward with a pleasant feeling on the face.
5. Avoid jerks in raising and lowering the trunk and the knees.

Results

This pose is a combination of the Cobra Pose and the Locust Pose. Muscles of the abdomen are stretched. It helps in digestion and improves the functioning of the internal viscera.

Discussion and References

Dhanuh means bow. Âsana means pose. Therefore, Dhanurâsana means Bow Pose (*Gh.S.* II, 18).

It resembles a stretched bow with a string.

Some teachers believe that it stimulates Maṇipur Cakra (solar plexus). Dhanurâsana of *Haṭha-Pradîpikâ* (I, 25) is not exactly the same as described in *Gh.S.* (II, 18).

We know a bow is used to shoot an arrow at a target. Here, symbolically, the bow is our body; Âtman (the Self) is the arrow; and Brahman is the target. Then, as the arrow, we become one with Brahman. "It (the target) is to be hit by a man who is not careless." (*M.U.* II, 2.4).

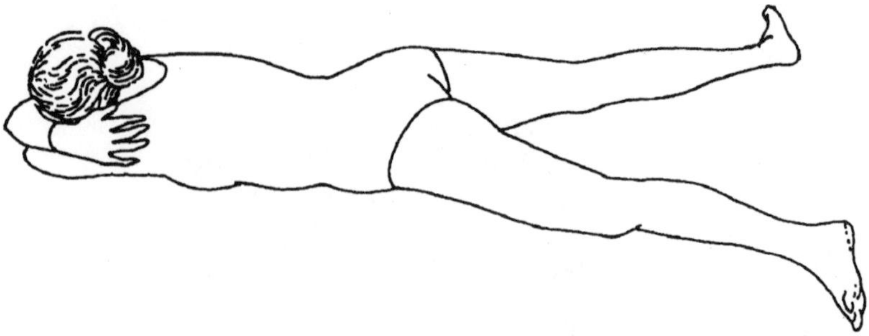

VI

MAKARÂSANA

Crocodile Pose

Technique

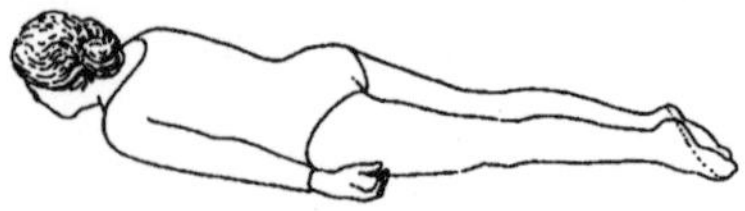

Lie prone, chin touching the ground, hands along the sides of the body.

Legs are stretched wide apart at a comfortable distance with toes pointing outward and heels facing each other.

Raise your chin.

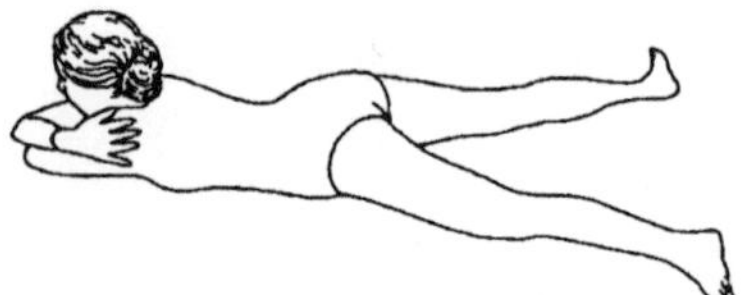

Now make triangles with your arms by placing elbows on each other and holding the shoulders by the hands. This makes the jaw of a crocodile (*Gh.S. II, 40)*.

Place your forehead on the stretched elbow triangle.

Relax and breathe rhythmically.

Suggestions

1. Point the toes outward and rotate the hip joints in such a way that the lower abdomen rests flatly on the ground.
2. When you make the triangles, place one hand under the armpit and the other hand over the armpit to grasp the shoulders.

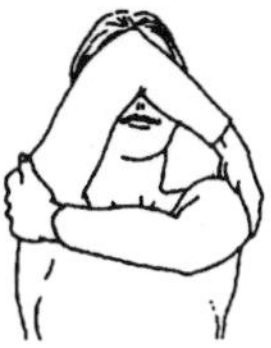

3. Breathe slowly, deeply, and smoothly.
4. Keep the duration of inhalation and exhalation as comfortable and equal as possible.

Results

It is a relaxation pose. The abdominal walls get massaged. It improves digestion. This pose is good for those who feel chilled relaxing on their backs. Overweight people may find this pose easier for relaxation.

Discussion and References

Makara means crocodile. Âsana means pose. Therefore, Makarâsana means Crocodile Pose (*Gh.S.* II, 40).

Lord Kṛṣṇa declares in *Šrîmadbhagavadgîtâ* (X, 31), "Of the aquatics, I am the crocodile."

The crocodile is selected as the greatest among creatures in the ocean, perhaps because it can live on the earth as well as in the water; perhaps also, because of its armour-like skin and long tapering jaws. It can also cross the ocean, which may be taken symbolically.

Crocodile is a carrier of Varuṇa Bîja (water seed) at Svâdhiṣṭhâna Cakra (hypogastric plexus), (*Ṣ.C.N.* 15).

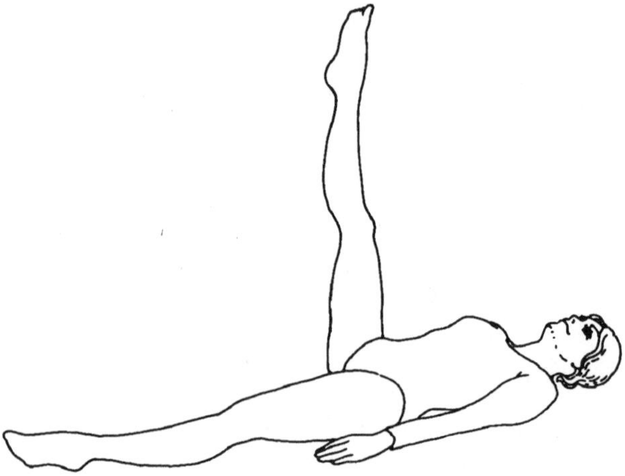

VII

ARDHA-HALÂSANA

Half-Plow Pose (First Stage)

Technique

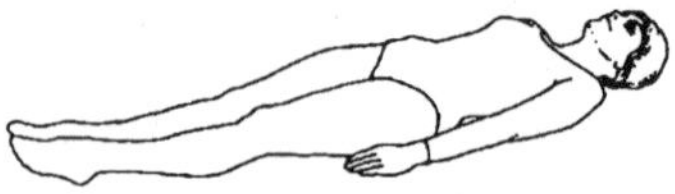

Lie supine, feet together, hands along the sides of the body, palms on the floor.

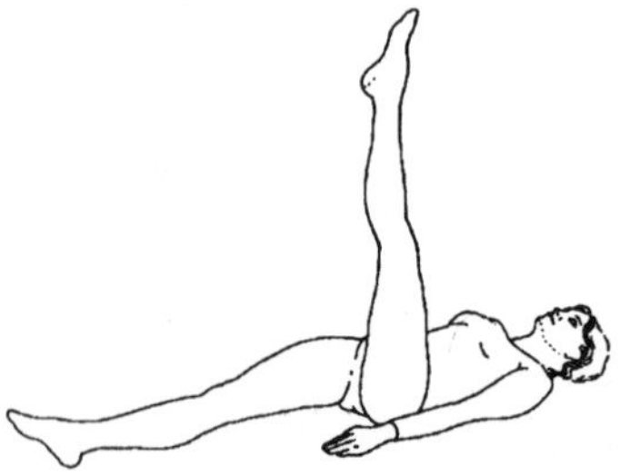

Raise your left leg slowly as far as you can go without bending your knee.

Hold for a few seconds and then come back to the original position slowly.

Now raise your right leg in the same manner, hold, and come back slowly.

Repeat three or four times.

Suggestions

1. Raise the leg slowly without jerks.
2. It can be done by maintaining the leg at an angle of 30° , 60° , and 90°.

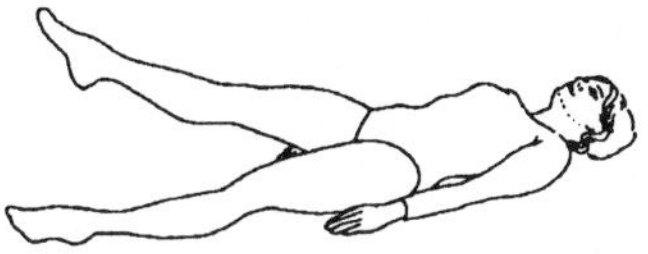

3. While coming down you may feel a sense of body disorientation or a disturbance of body image, as if your foot is not landing in the same place as it began. It is all right, and will disappear in due course of time.

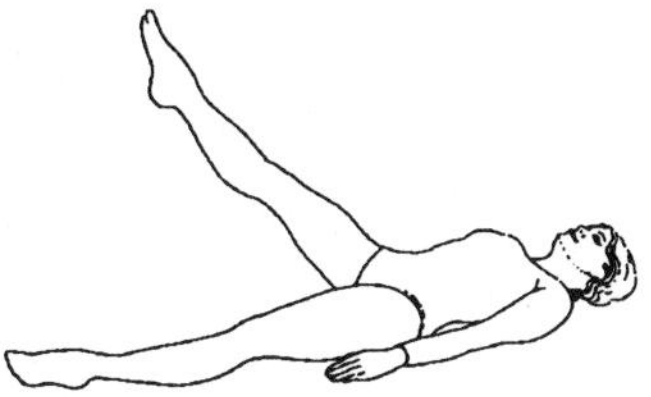

4. Keep stretching the legs while lifting them. Be careful that the stretch doesn't give a sense of uneasiness or a cramp.

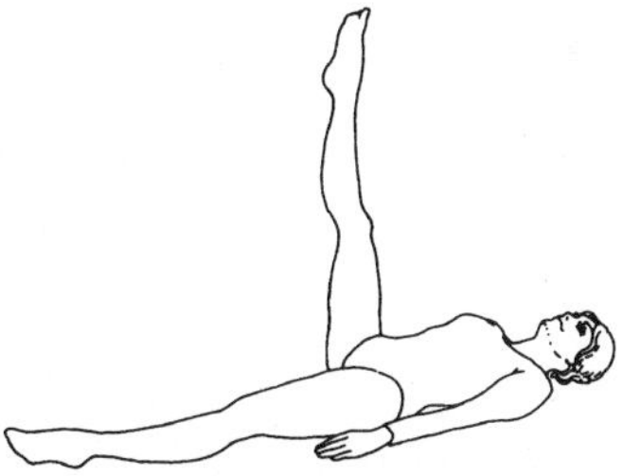

Results

It prepares a student to practice Halâsana (Plow Pose). It increases the circulation in the lower extremities and helps to strengthen the thigh and abdominal muscles.

Discussion and References

Ardha means half. Hala means plow of the traditional wooden type used in India. Âsana means pose. Therefore, Ardha-Halâsana means Half-Plow Pose.

Here, we have outlined the first stage, in which only one leg is raised at a time.

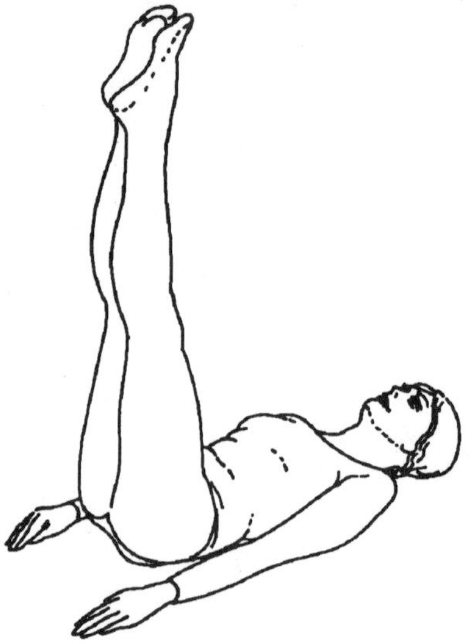

VIII

ARDHA-HALÂSANA+

Half-Plow Pose (Second Stage)

Technique

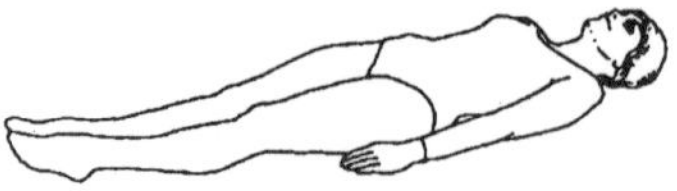

Lie supine, feet together, hands along the sides of the body, palms on the ground.

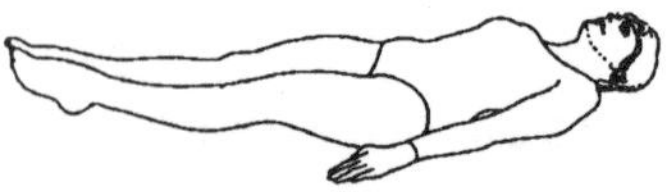

After practicing the first stage of Ardha-Halâsana, raise both legs together without bending the knees, and hold at a 15° angle from the floor.

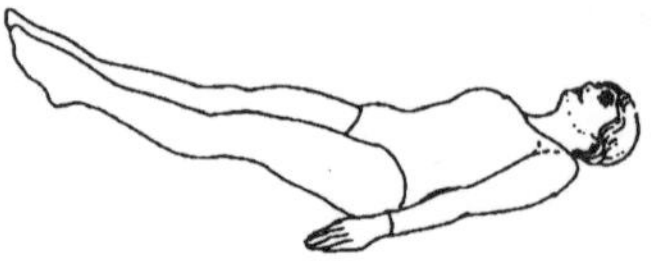

Then raise further to 30° and hold; then raise up to 45° and hold; then to 60° and hold; and then go up to 90° and hold.

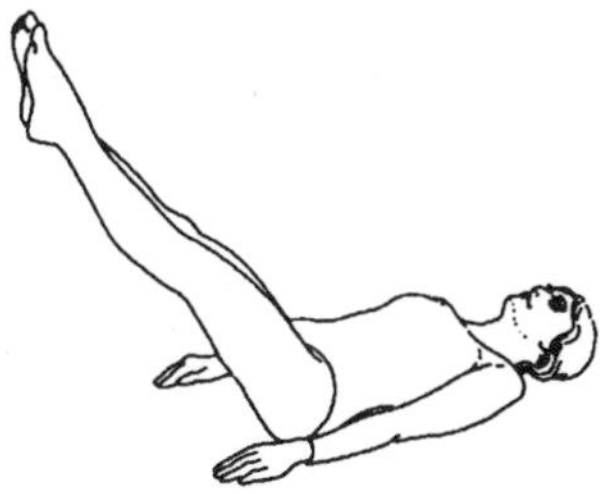

Come back to the original position in the reverse manner by holding at 60°, 45°, 30°, and 15°.

Suggestions

1. Raise legs slowly without jerks or bending the knees.
2. Maintain the pose at each angle for a few seconds.
3. Those who have weak abdominal muscles may find the pose difficult. They should be patient and forego maintaining the position at uncomfortable angles.

Results

It secures the health of the abdomen by strengthening the abdominal viscera, helps in digestion, and works against constipation.

Discussion and References

See discussion on Halâsana. Because both legs are included, this is considered the second stage of the Half-Plow.

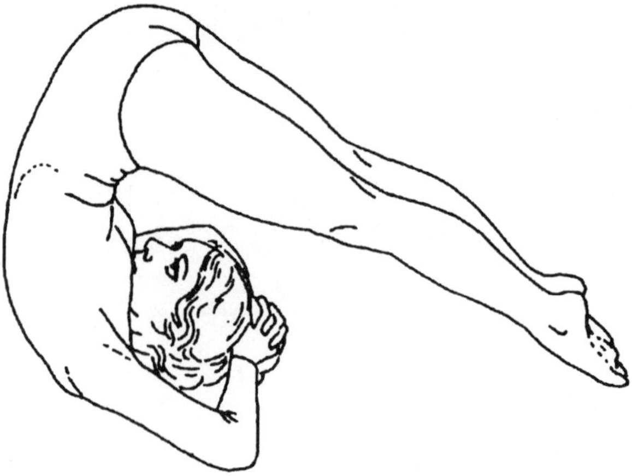

IX
HALÂSANA
Plow Pose

Technique

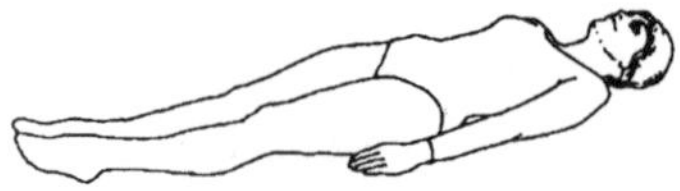

Lie supine with feet together, hands along the sides of the body, and palms on the floor.

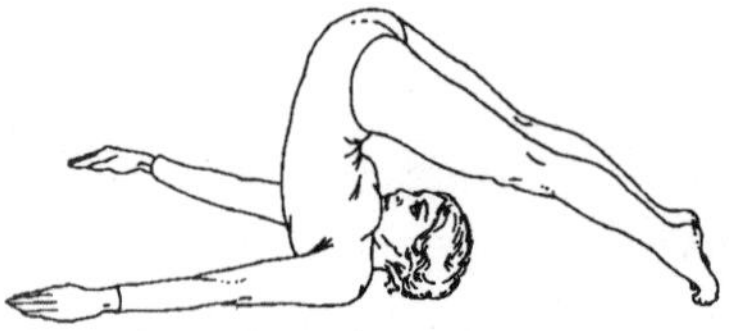

After the practice of Ardha-Halâsana both first and second stages, raise the legs further and place the toes beyond your head.

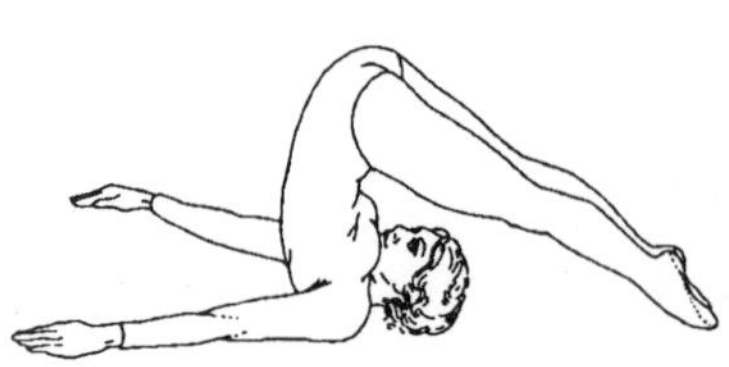

Keep toes together and stretched. Palms remain in the original position firmly on the floor.

Maintain the position for some time and then push your toes farther beyond your head.

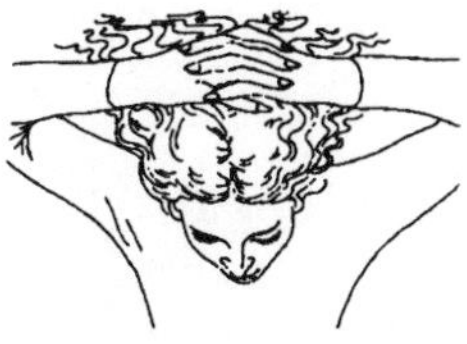

Now bring your hands around your head and form a finger lock, then push your toes further.

Suggestions

1. This pose is done gradually without jerks by shifting the pressure from the lumbo-sacral part to the lower dorsal, upper dorsal, and cervical parts of the spine.

2. If you find difficulty in the beginning because of a stiff spine, be satisfied with whatever position you can remain in comfortably.

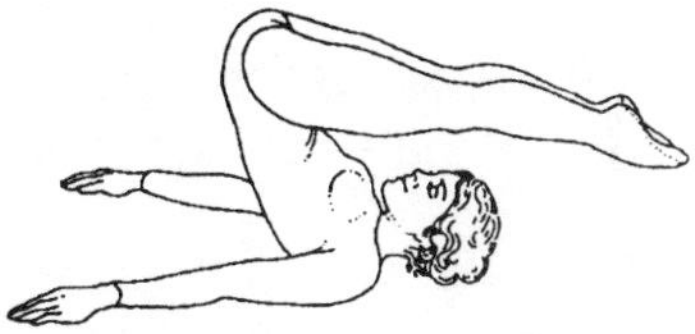

3. The finger lock around the head is only formed after the toes have touched the floor.

4. The legs may shake. In that case, a slight bend of the knees is allowed.

Results

It contributes to the suppleness of the body by maintaining the elasticity of the spinal column. It helps in developing the abdominal muscles. The pose prevents constipation, improves digestion, and also influences the glands situated in the viscera, such as the adrenals.

Discussion and References

Halâsana means Plow Pose because it resembles an Indian plow.

As a plow makes the land fertile, in the same way this pose may enhance fertility and vitality.

It also seems that Plow Pose is a good exercise to strengthen the lower part of the body for raising the Kuṇḍalinî. Perhaps this is related to the fact that Âkâša Tattva (ether element), situated at the throat, has "ha" as its seed and presiding deity as Sadâšiva. Concentrating on that opens the gate of liberation, and it also resists the aging process (*Gh.S.* III, 80-81 and *Ṣ.C.N.* 13 & 31).

Pṛthvî Tattva (the element of earth), located at the perineum, has "la" as its seed, and Brahmâ, the Creator, as its presiding deity. Concentration on that makes a person steady (*Gh.S.* III, 70).

Therefore, Halâsana provides stability, health, and at the same time opens the gate for higher experiences.

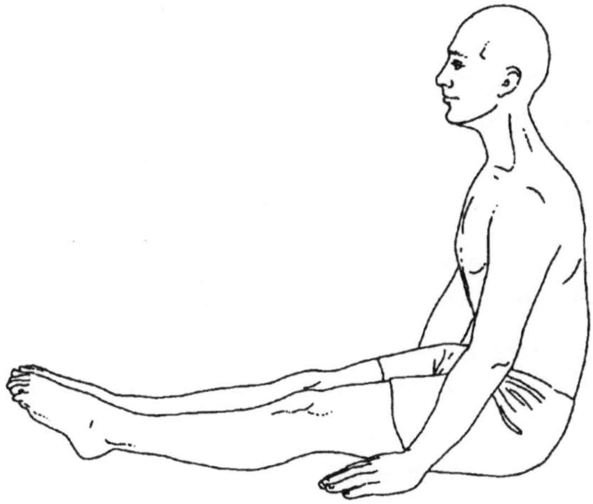

X

DAṆḌÂSANA

Stick Pose

Technique

Lie supine with the feet together, hands along the sides of the body, and palms on the floor.

Sit up slowly, with your legs remaining extended and palms on the floor. Close your eyes. Maintain the pose for some time and then return to the original position.

Repeat two or three times.

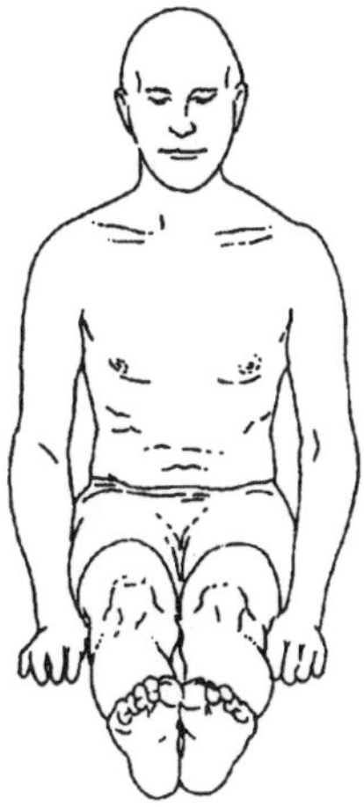

Suggestions

1. Gradually lift your head and body to a sitting condition without jerking or using the support of your elbows.

2. Rest the palms lightly on the ground without using them to support your weight.

Results

It contributes to the suppleness of the body by tensing and relaxing the body. It is helpful in reducing excess fat in the thighs and abdomen. It may serve as a meditative pose for those who cannot bend or cross their legs.

Discussion and References

Daṇḍa means stick. Âsana means pose. Therefore, Daṇḍâsana means Stick Pose.

To sit like the stick indicates a stability both physical and mental, which may result in a higher experience.

Traditionally, this pose is mentioned by Vyâsa in the commentary on Patañjali's *Yoga Sûtras*, II, 46. It is explained by Vâcasapati in his commentary on Vyâsa's work.

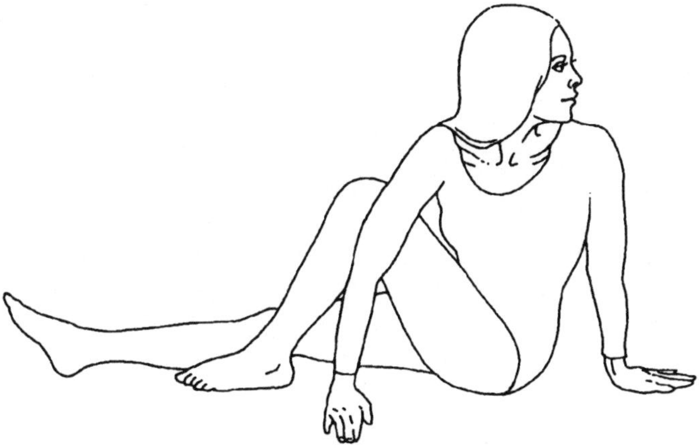

XI
VAKRÂSANA
Twist Pose

Technique

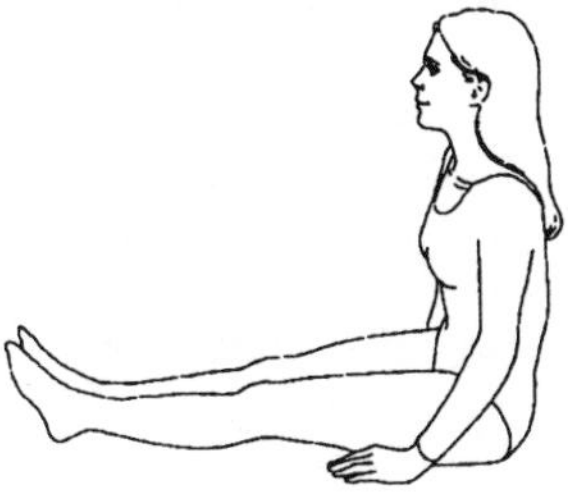

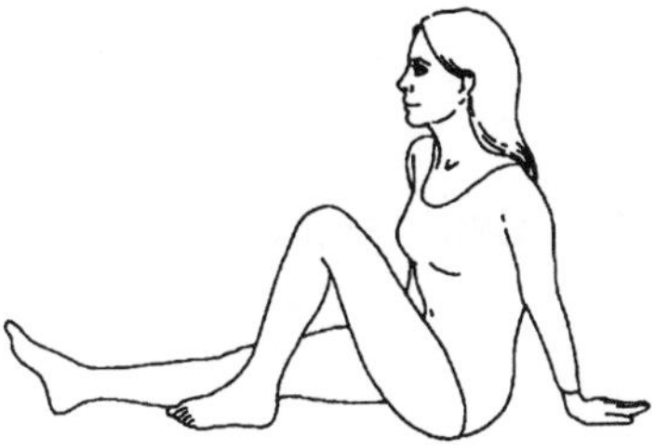

Sit in Daṇḍâsana (Stick Pose).

Raise your left knee and place the left foot next to the stretched right knee.

Place your left palm behind you in the line of your spine, with fingers pointing outward and together in such a way that the body remains as straight as possible.

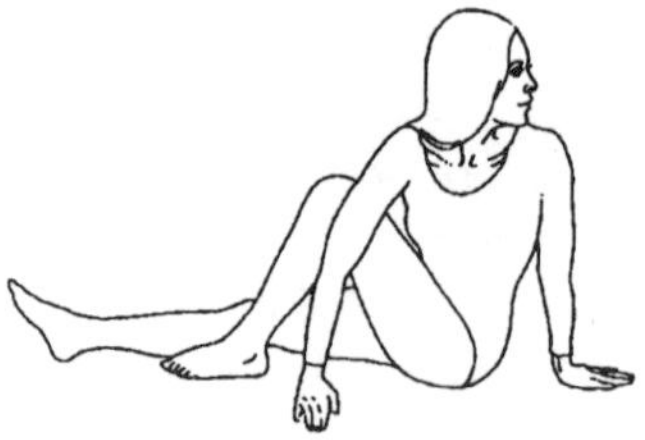

After crossing your right arm over your raised left knee, place the palm on the ground, fingers pointing to the left.

Twist your trunk to the left and look behind you as far as possible.

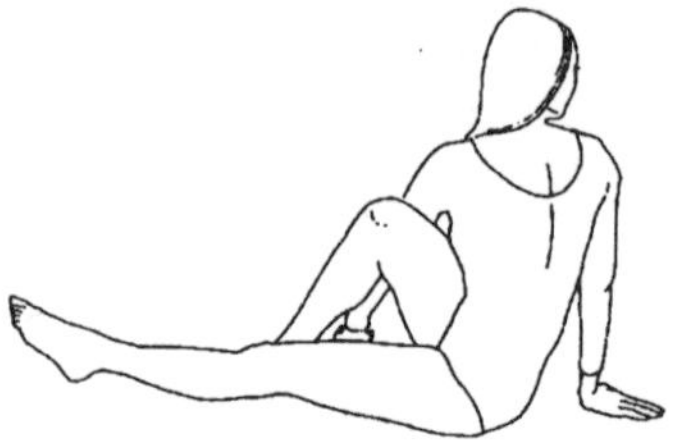

Release in reverse order and switch to the other side.

Repeat and then relax.

Suggestions

1. Place your foot next to the knee and keep your trunk as erect as possible.
2. Try to keep your knee straight, even if this means not touching the floor with your hand.
3. Keep your elbow straight, palm in the line of the spine with fingers pointing outward.
4. When you switch from one side to the other, do it slowly.

Results

It makes the nervous system healthy. The abdominal area, neck and eyes also get exercise.

Discussion and References

Vakra means twist. Âsana means pose. Therefore, Vakrâsana means Twist Pose.

As the standard Matsyendrâsana is difficult to assume, Ardha-Matyendrâsana is proposed. However, it is also difficult in many cases. Therefore, Vakrâsana was introduced to Yoga discipline by Swâmî Kuvalayânanda (*Âsanas*, p.83), as an easier exercise preparatory to Ardha-Matsyendrâsana.

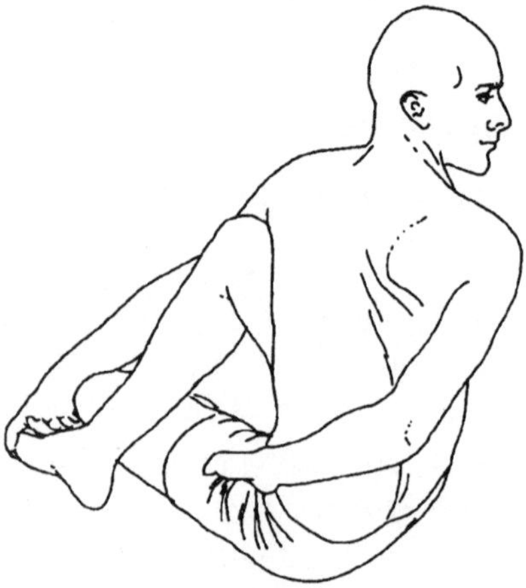

XII

ARDHA-MATSYENDRÂSANA

Half-Matsyendra Pose

Technique

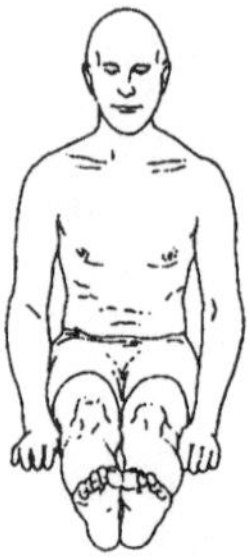

Sit. Extend your legs in front in Daṇḍâsana (Stick Pose).

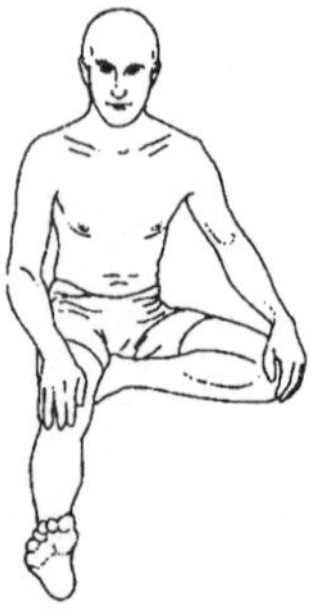

Bend your left leg at the knee and place the heel at the perineum (between the anus and genitals).

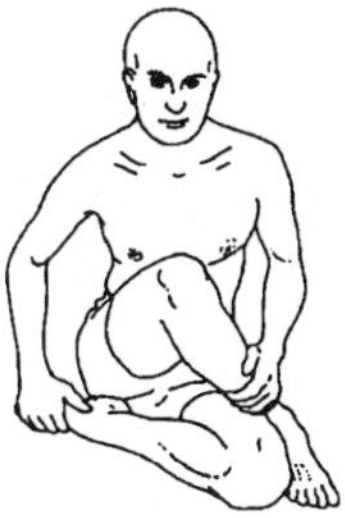

Lift your right foot and place it at the left side of the left knee.

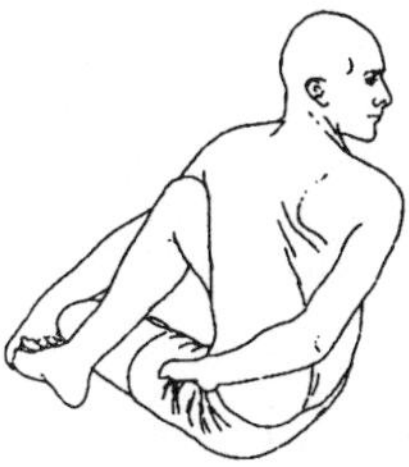

Raise your left arm, take it around the right knee and catch hold of your right big toe, elbow facing toward the right knee.

Catch your left thigh with the right hand by reaching behind your back; look beyond your right shoulder.

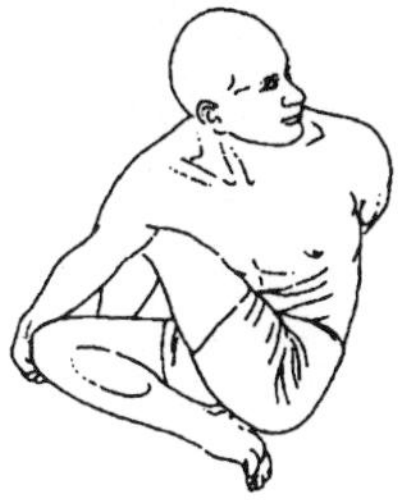

Hold the pose for some time. Release this pose systematically and repeat on the other side.

Suggestions

1. Be aware of the touch of the heel at the perineum, as it generally slips.
2. Try to keep the trunk erect.
3. Keep one knee flat on the floor, and the cross-over knee upright.
4. Look as far back as possible.
5. Use an index finger hook to catch your big toe.

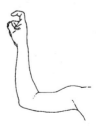

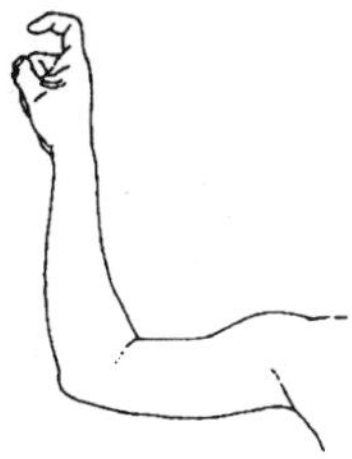

Results

It improves digestion and removes constipation. It maintains the health of the spine. It helps in awakening the Kuṇḍalinî.

Discussion and References

This pose is a simplification of Matsyendrâsana, named after the great ancient exponent of Haṭha Yoga, Šrî Matsyendra Nâth.

In this pose, as the heel touches the perineum, it is evident that it will stimulate Mulâdhâra Cakra and consequently awaken the Kuṇḍalinî.

The twist of the spine may help the arousal. Not only that, it will regulate the nostril breathing.

In the traditional Matsyendrâsana, the foot is placed on top of the thigh, rather than at the perineum, which has a wider effect on the abdominal viscera (*H.P.* I, 26-27).

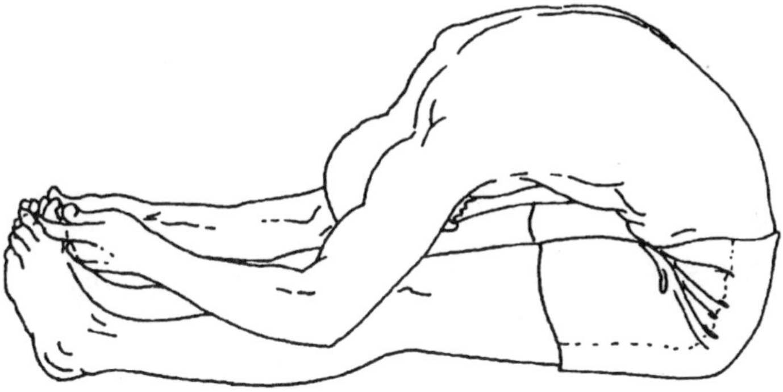

XIII
PAŠCIMATÂNÂSANA
Posterior Stretch Pose

Technique

Lie supine with feet together, hands along the sides of the body, and palms on the floor. Sit up gradually, as you do in the Stick Pose.

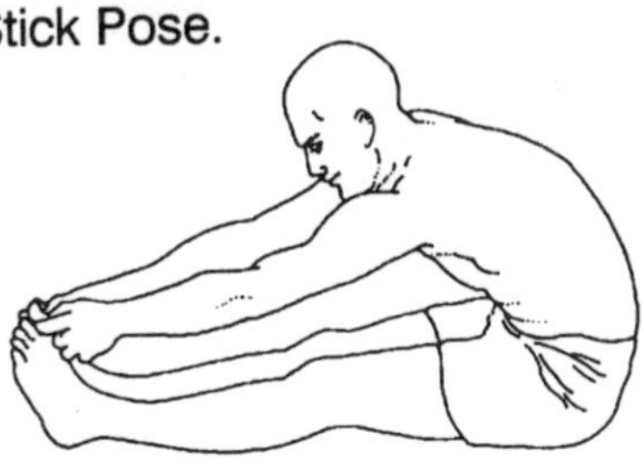

Now, slowly bring your hands near your toes by bending forward.

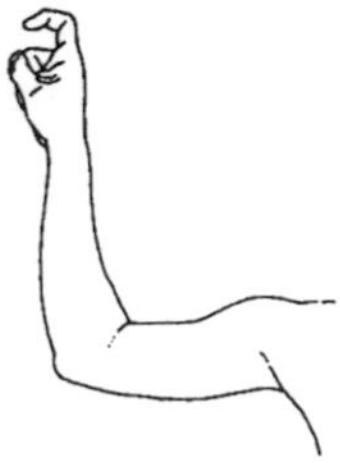

Catch hold of your big toes by forming finger hooks with your index fingers; left index finger hooking the left toe, and right index finger hooking the right toe.

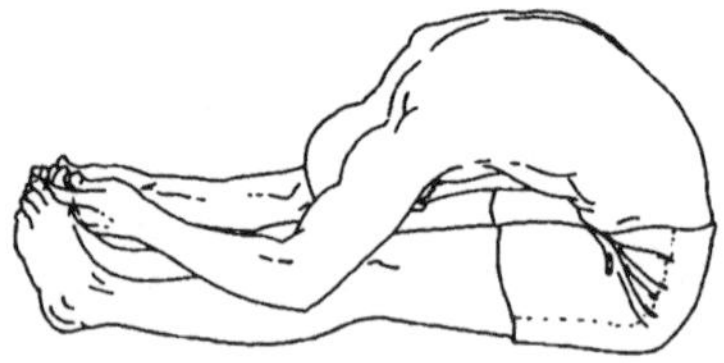

Do not bend or raise your knees. After securing the position, bend forward and place your forehead on the knees. Maintain the pose for some time and slowly come back to a sitting position.

Repeat two or three times and then relax in Šavâsana (Corpse Pose).

Suggestions

1. Keep your knees straight.
2. If you cannot catch hold of your toes, hold your ankles or even your knees.
3. Avoid jerking or bouncing the legs on the floor.
4. Do not hold this pose for long periods, without proper instruction from a teacher.
5. As you become more flexible, you may form a finger lock around your soles instead of catching your big toes. (See Halâsana for the illustration of this finger lock.)

Results

This pose secures the health of the whole body. It is a fine posterior stretch; at the same time, it contracts the anterior parts of the body, particularly the abdominal region. Thus, it provides health for the nervous, circulatory, digestive, excretive, and procreative systems. It is very useful in helping a student of the spiritual path by arousing Kuṇḍalinî Šakti and making him aware of a subtle sound.

Discussion and References

Paščima means back. Tâna means stretch. Âsana means pose. Therefore, Paščimatânâsana means Posterior Stretch Pose.

Paščima also indicates Suṣumṇâ (the spinal nerve), through which latent energy ascends.

This posture, therefore, works on two Cakras in the body. It seems to stimulate the lower Cakras first, and then the higher Cakras.

It is referred to in *Gh.S.* (II, 26) as Paščimottânâsana. Uttâna also means stretch.

In *Š.S.* III, 110-112, the same pose is described by the name Ugrâsana. Others, however, consider this to be a different pose.

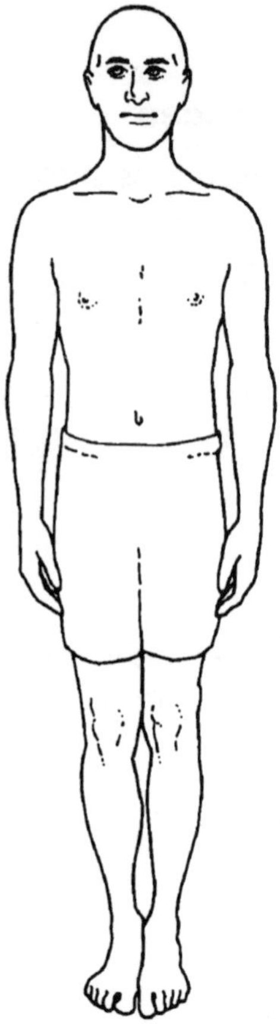

XIV

STAMBHÂSANA

Pillar Pose

Technique

Stand straight, feet together, hands along the sides of the body.

Maintain the position for some time.

Then close your eyes and continue to stand, remaining as stable as possible.

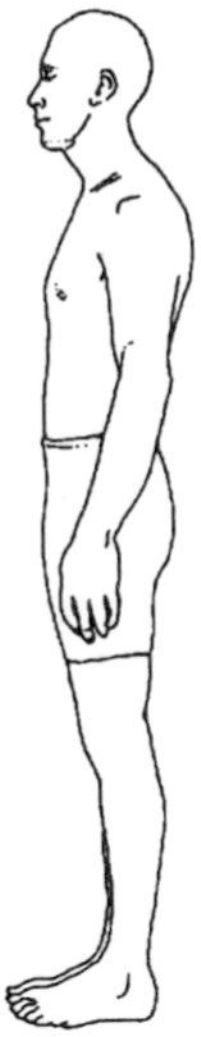

Suggestions

1. Keep your toes and heels together.
2. Maintain the erectness of the body.
3. Once you close your eyes, do not open them again while holding the pose.
4. You may feel some swaying of the body in any direction. It generally happens, though not always in the same direction.

Results

It helps in increasing will power if the student resists the sway, and improves the balance mechanism. It makes a person aware of his body rhythms.

Discussion and References

Stambha means pillar. Âsana means pose. Therefore, Stambhâsana means Pillar Pose.

A pillar is a symbol of stability and an important part of any foundation.

This pose was introduced by SKY Foundation in order to make students aware of the effects of finer forces or imagination on the posture.

If the student imagines that he is swaying forward, backward, sideways, or in a circular pattern – the body will actually move accordingly, in most cases.

This pose may be used to test suggestibility, and to observe the effects of Tattvas in the body.

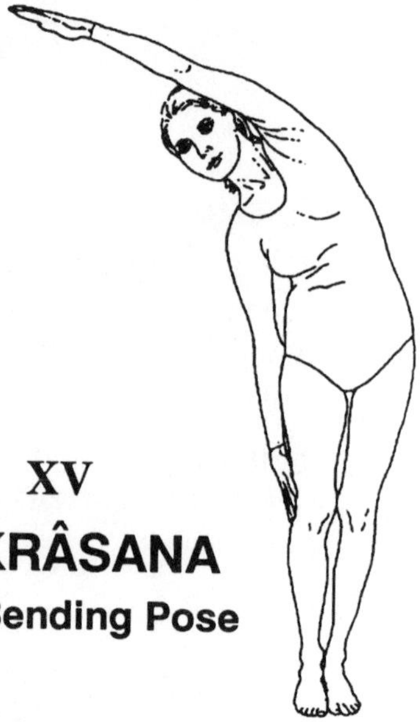

XV
CAKRÂSANA
Side-Bending Pose

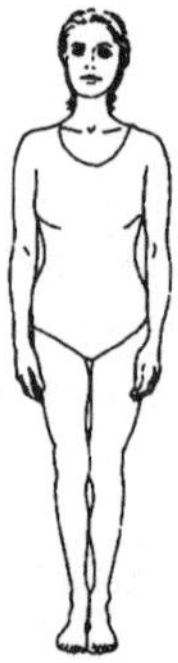

Technique

Stand with feet together, toes together, and hands along the sides of the body.

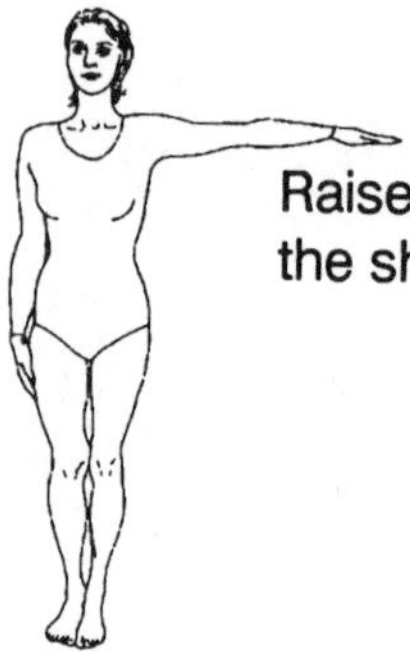

Raise the left arm slowly until it comes to the line of the shoulders.

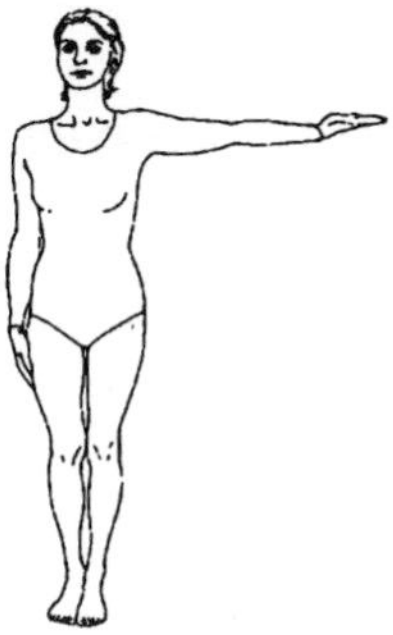

Turn the palm up and bring your arm up to your left ear, keeping it straight.

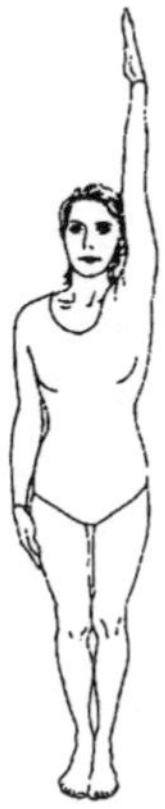

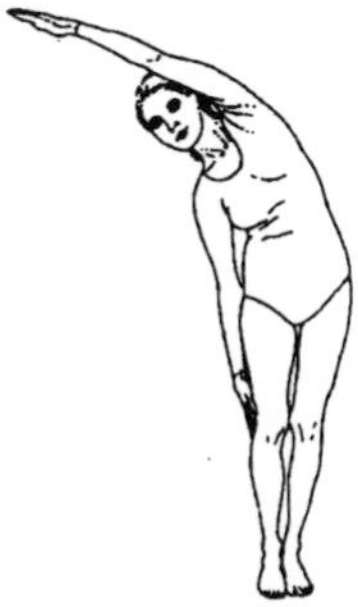

Now bend to the right and hold for some time. Come back slowly to the original standing position.

Repeat with the right arm in the same way. Raise the right arm to the shoulder line and turn the palm up. Go further up to the ear and then bend to the left side. Hold for some time and return to the original standing position slowly.

Repeat three times.

Suggestions

1. While bending, keep your head and arm together, without bending the neck and keeping the arm straight and stretched.
2. Look ahead, in the line of your eyes.
3. Don't bring your hip out in order to get the curve.
4. Keep your feet close together.

Results

It gives the spine a lateral stretch, and adds to the health of the abdominal viscera. It increases the circulation in the upper extremities with a feeling of blood flow in the arms; and, in general, it tones the spine.

Discussion and References

This is a modern and easy variation introduced by Swâmî Kuvalayânanda (1883-1966) in order to provide a lateral stretch for the spine, which generally is not found in classical poses. The traditional Cakrâsana (*V.U.* V, 15 & 17), is quite different from the Cakrâsana described here.

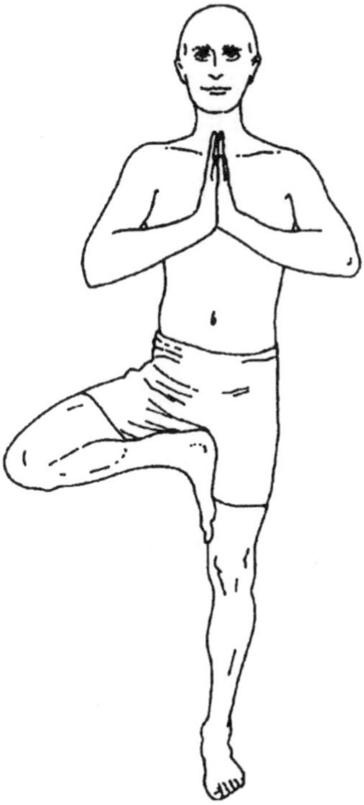

XVI

VṚKṢÂSANA

Tree Pose

Technique

Stand with heels and toes together, hands along the sides of the body.

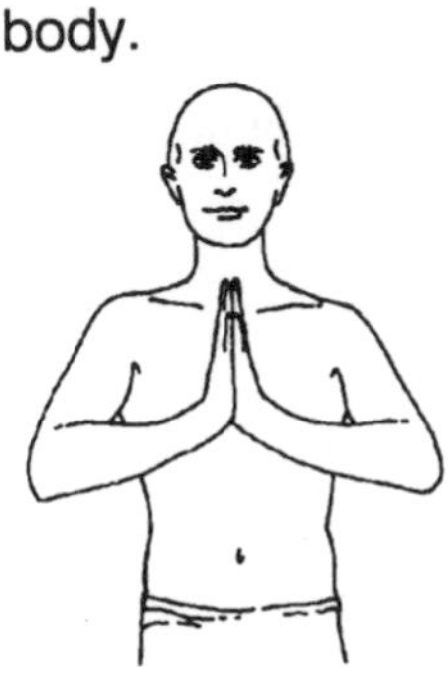

Place your hands in front of the chest in Namaskâra Mudrâ (Indian way of salutation).

Now raise your left leg and place the foot at the right thigh, heel near the hip joint, sole touching the inside of the thigh.

Beginners may use their hand to place their foot. Keep the body erect.

Hold the pose for some time and switch to the other leg. Repeat two or three times.

Hold the pose with closed eyes as well.

Suggestions

1. Keep the body straight and the knee pointing to the side, not toward the front or back.
2. Try to bring your foot to the thigh without the help of your hand.
3. Fix your gaze at any stable point at eye level.
4. Fix your gaze at an imaginary point when you try the pose with closed eyes.

Results

It helps in training a person to focus attention and develop will power.

Discussion and References

Vṛkṣa means tree. Âsana means pose. Therefore,Vṛkṣâsana means Tree Pose.

A tree gives fruits without discrimination and without keeping them to itself.

When the tree is full of fruit, it bends.

In the same way, when the Yoga student achieves some fruits of his practices, he becomes humble and shares his fruit with others. If this idea occurs during Yogic practices and lingers on, it will have a positive effect on the aspirant's day-to-day behavior.

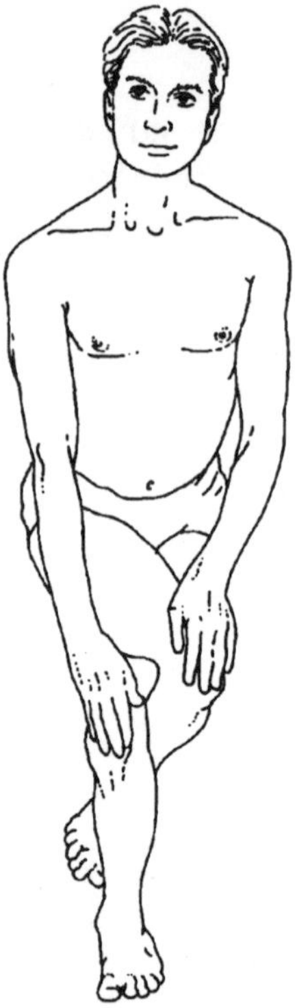

XVII

SAṄKAṬÂSANA

Difficult Pose

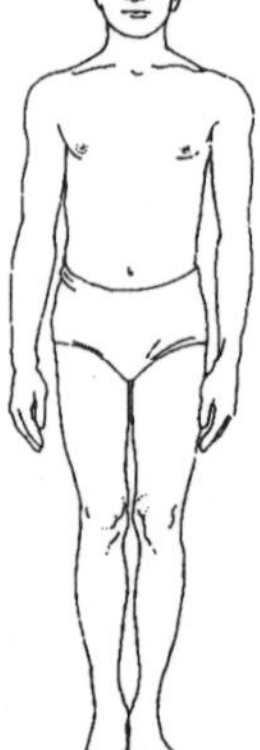

Technique

Stand with your feet together, toes together, and hands along the sides of the body.

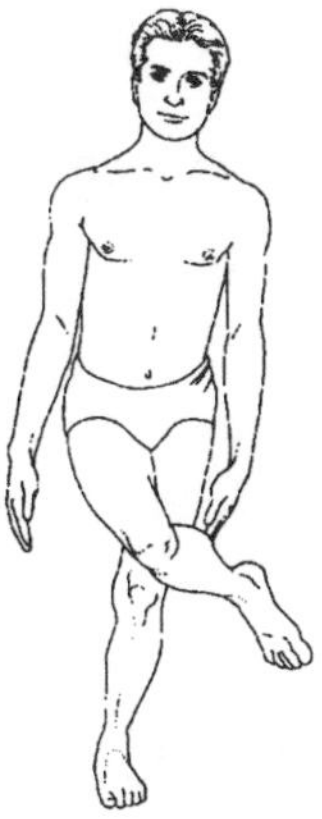

Raise your right leg, bend the left leg, and then encircle and tuck the right leg around the left.

Place your palms on the opposite knees.

Hold the pose for some time, and then come back to the original position.

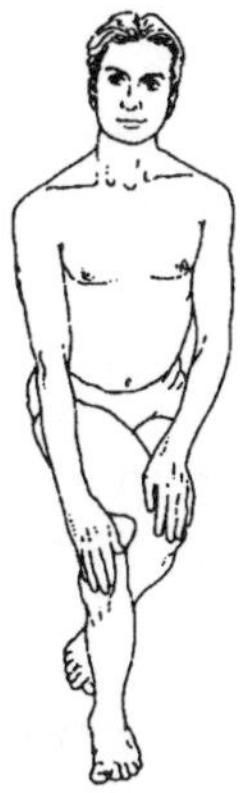

Repeat the pose with the left leg and relax.

Suggestions

1. It is easier to encircle the leg by raising the other leg a bit higher.
2. Avoid jerks.
3. Place your hands on the opposite knees; that is, right hand on the left knee and left hand on the right knee.
4. Be as erect as possible.
5. Fix your gaze. This will aid in balancing.
6. It is difficult for those people who have heavy thighs. They are requested to be satisfied by lifting the leg and maintaining balance – not by excluding the pose because they cannot do it.
7. This pose is easier to practice standing on a hard surface, rather than on a soft surface.
8. If you find the pose difficult, try lying on your back instead of standing, as encircling the legs is easier in a lying position.

Results

It increases attention and will power. It makes the nervous system healthy. It helps to shape the thighs.

Discussion and References

In Sanskrit, Saṅkaṭa means difficult. Âsana means pose. Therefore, Saṅkaṭâsana means Difficult Pose *(Gh.S. II, 28).*

Generally people find it easier to practice such poses on one side of their body rather than the other. That is because one side is dominant.

Gradually it can be done with eyes closed, but it is not necessary in the beginning, as it is difficult. Open eyes help in balance and stability.

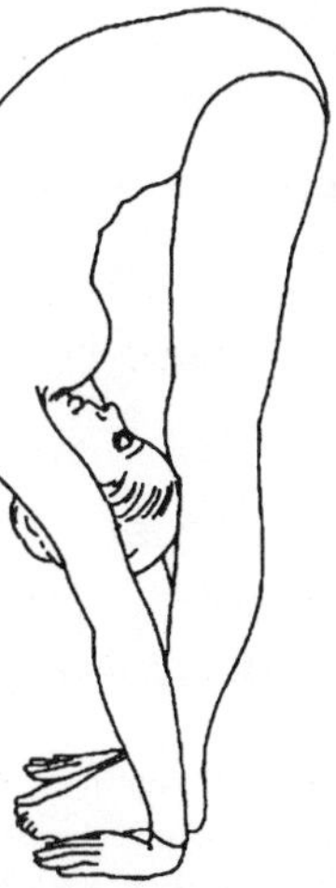

XVIII
PÂDAHASTÂSANA
Hand-to-Foot Pose

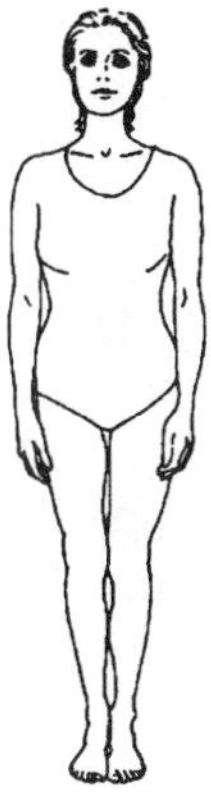

Technique

Stand with heels and toes together, and hands along the sides of the body.

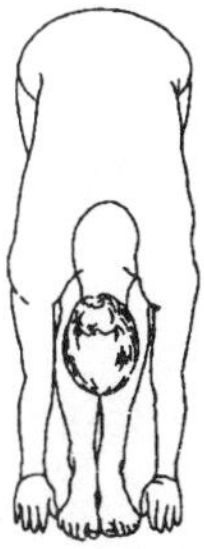

Slowly bring both of your hands toward your feet by bending your body at the waist without bending your knees.

Place both hands by the sides of your feet, palms touching the floor and fingers pointing forward.

Be steady.

Bring your forehead toward the knees and maintain it for some time.

Now bring your head up, take your hands off the floor, and stand erect, with hands by your sides.

Repeat the pose three or four times.

Suggestions

1. Keep your feet together.
2. Before you bring your forehead to the knees, be sure of your balance.
3. Do not bend your knees.
4. Avoid jerks both in bringing your head to the knees and your hands to the ground.
5. Do it slowly and gradually.

Results

It improves digestion, increases the blood circulation in the upper parts of the body, tones the nervous system, and strengthens the leg muscles.

Discussion and References

Pâda means foot. Hasta means hand. Âsana means pose. Therefore, Pâdahastâsana means Hand-to-Foot Pose.

This pose is not described in any authentic traditional text, per se. However, it seems to be a variation of the Posterior Stretch, with a shift of the center of gravity.

People who find the Posterior Stretch difficult may practice this first with benefit.

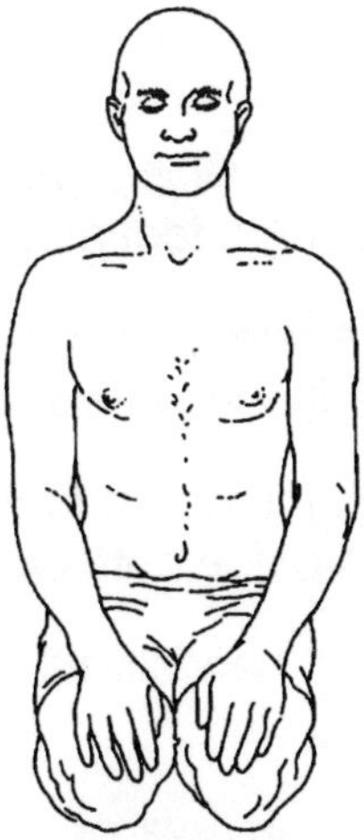

XIX
VAJRÂSANA
Pelvic Pose

Technique

Assume Daṇḍâsana (Stick Pose).

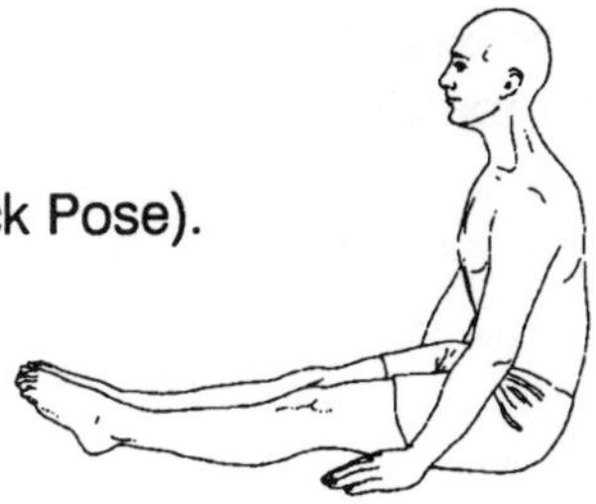

Bend the left leg at the knee. Grasp your left ankle with the left hand and place the foot near the buttock, keeping the heel outward.

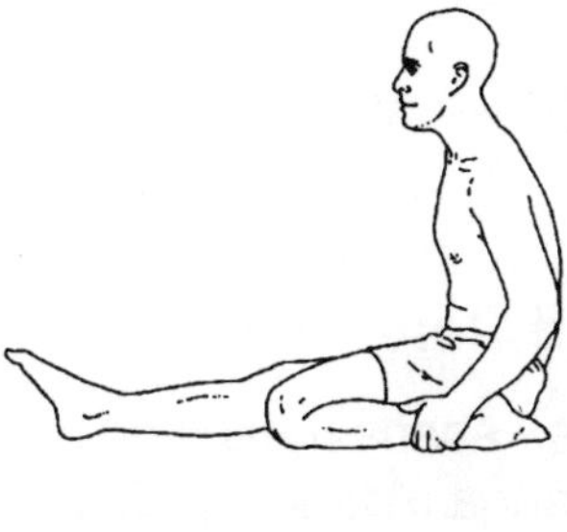

Now take the support of the left hand and lean slightly on the left side by sitting on the left sole.

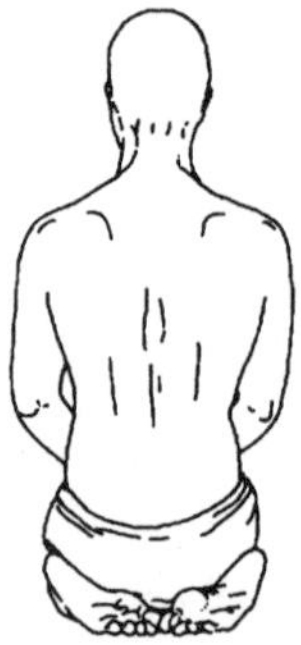

Bend your right leg, grasp the right ankle, and place the right foot near the right buttock.

Now sit straight on your inner soles, toes touching, keeping the heels out.

Or, sit on the ground with the feet just touching the sides of the buttocks.

Place your hands on the knees. Close your eyes.

Sit for some time and release in reverse order.

Suggestions

1. Sit erect and do not sit on the heels.

2. In the beginning, place your palms on the floor while you are sitting on your soles, to help support your weight. This will prevent injury to knees or ankle joints, particularly for those who have stiff joints.

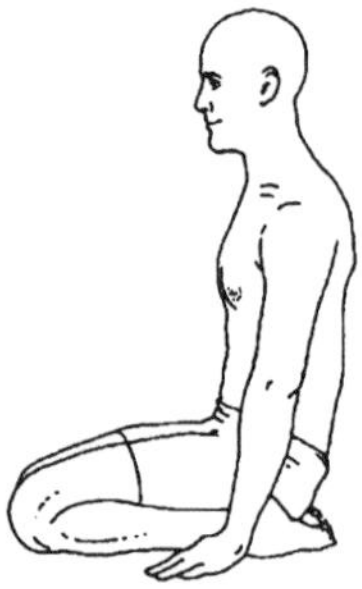

Results

It improves digestion, tones the pelvic region, and helps in meditation.

Discussion and References

Vajra means penis. Âsana means pose. A free rendering by Swâmî Kuvalayânanda (*Âsanas*, p. 87) is Pelvic Pose (*Gh.S.* II, 12).

Siddhâsana is also known as Vajrâsana (*H.P.* I, 37 and *Y.K.U.* I, 4-6), which has a different technique. The name Vajrâ is also the name of the Nâdî which runs inside the Suṣumṇâ (Spinal Cord), (*Ṣ.C.N.*).

This pose seems to be of Buddhist origin. It is a popular pose for Zazen.

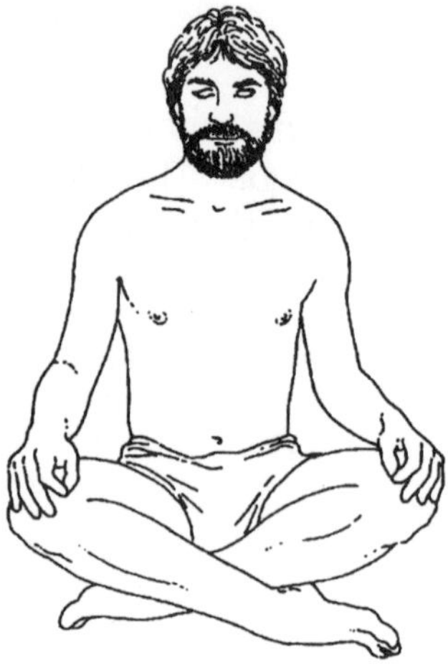

XX
SUKHÂSANA
Easy Pose

Technique

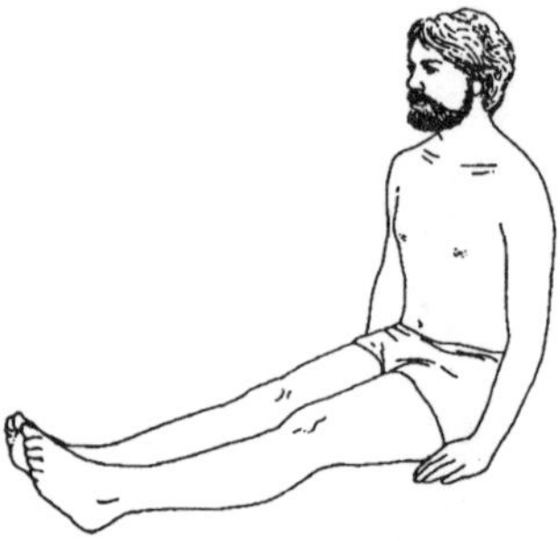

Assume Daṇḍâsana (Stick Pose).

Bend the left leg and place the foot under your right thigh; place the right foot under the left thigh.

Place your hands on the knees.

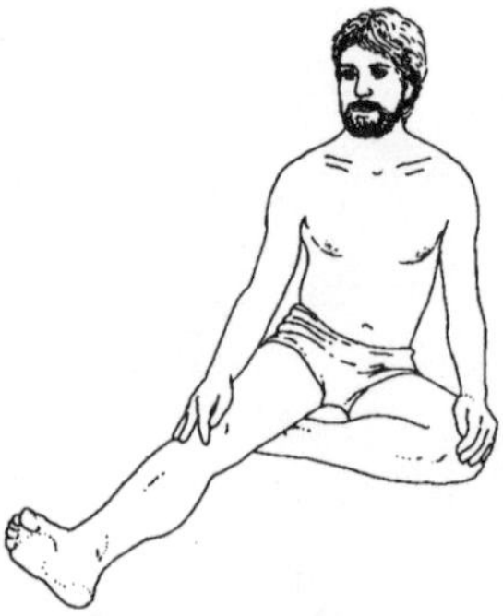

Sit erect with the spine, neck and head in a balanced condition.

Close your eyes, or fix your gaze at the tip of your nose.

Suggestions

1. Keep the spine, neck, and head in a balanced, erect condition.
2. When you are sitting, try to bring your feet under the thighs, but don't force. The important aspect of the pose is the erect, balanced condition of the body with comfort.

Results

It is an easy meditative pose. It increases the blood supply in the pelvic region, and slows the respiration and metabolic rates. It removes congestion in the internal viscera.

Discussion and References

Sukha means easy or comfortable. Âsana means pose. Sukhâsana, therefore, means Easy Pose.

This is popularly known as tailor's seat, so far as the lower extremities are concerned.

Patañjali does not describe any particular technical pose used by Haṭha Yoga. He does mention, however, the quality of a pose as steady, stable, easy, and comfortable (*P.Y.S.* II, 46).

In the commentary of Vyâsa, Sukhâsana is included as one of the poses. *Daršanopaniṣad* (III, 12-13) states: "In whichever manner comfort and courage are produced, that is known as Sukhâsana; a weak man should adopt such posture."

And in the Mantra section of *Trišikhibrâhmṇopaniṣad* (51-52), "That – wherein comfort and steadiness are attained somehow or other – is known as the Sukhâsana."

It is useful to mention that in Padmâsana (Lotus Pose), both feet are on the thighs; in Vîrâsana (Hero Pose), one is on the thigh, the other underneath; in Sukhâsana (Easy Pose), both are under or near the thighs. It depends on gradual training to finally develop Padmâsana and Baddha Padmâsana (Bound Lotus).

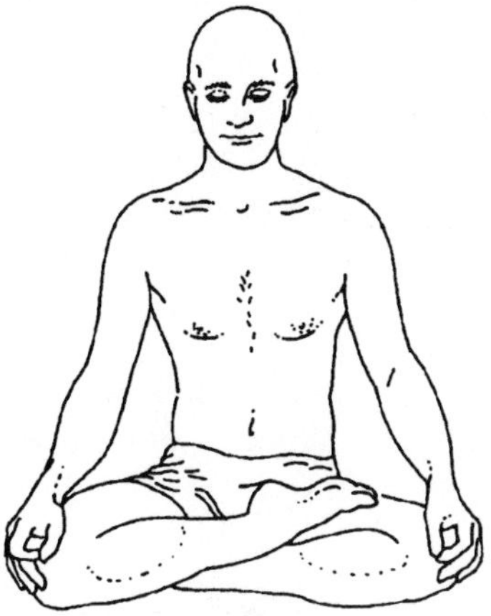

XXI
VÎRÂSANA
Hero Pose

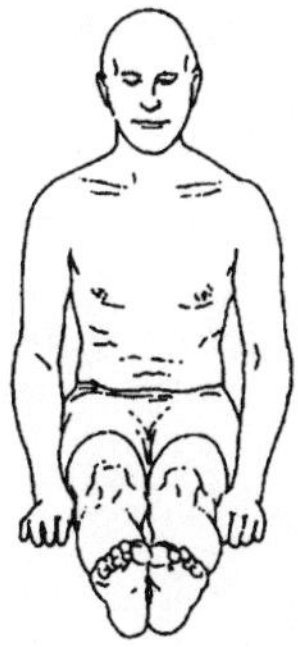

Technique

Assume Daṇḍâsana (Stick Pose).

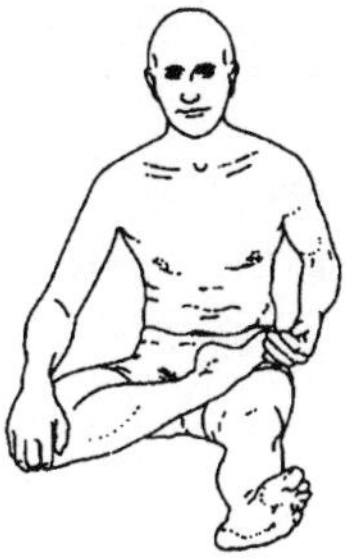

Fold your right leg at the knee and place it on the left thigh.

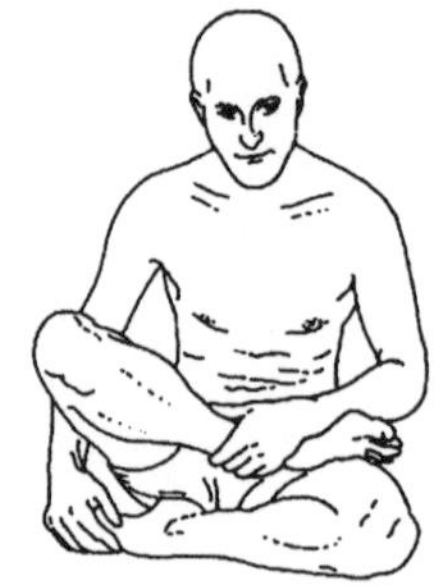

Put the left foot under the right thigh.

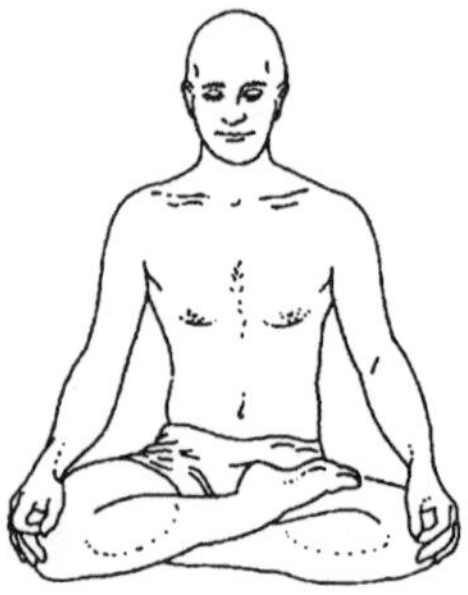

Keep your hands on the knees in Jñâna Mudrâ.*

Keep your eyes closed or keep the eyes in a nasal gaze.

Maintain the pose as long as you feel comfortable and then release.

Suggestions

1. Keep your spine, neck, and head erect and in a balanced condition.
2. Increase the duration gradually.
3. Try to keep your knees touching the floor.

Results

It has the advantage of a meditative pose. It is easier than Padmâsana and may be considered a preliminary practice for the Lotus Pose for those with stiff knees.

Discussion and References

Vîra means hero. Âsana means pose. Therefore, Vîrâsana means Hero Pose.

This pose is described in *H.P.* I, 21.

Gh.S. II, 17 describes this pose with slight variation.

Vîra also means alert. Therefore, Vîrâsana may lead to an alert condition.

This is also known as Ardha-Padmâsana, the Half-Lotus Pose.

**Jñâna Mudrâ (Symbol of Knowledge), is performed by touching the tip of the index finger with the thumb of the same hand and keeping the palms and the other three fingers comfortably stretched.*

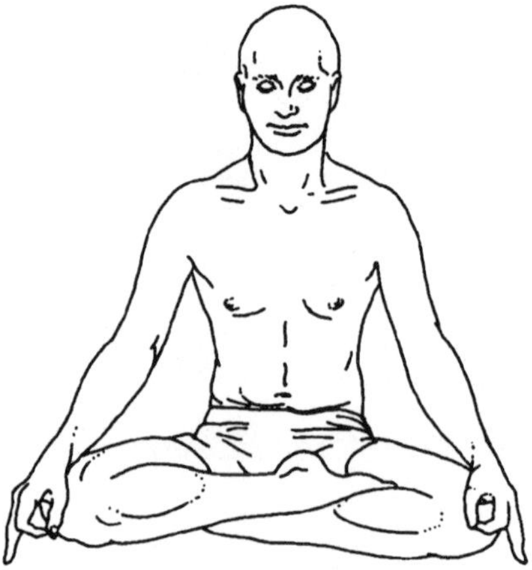

XXII
SVASTIKÂSANA
Auspicious Pose

Technique

Assume Daṇḍâsana (Stick Pose).

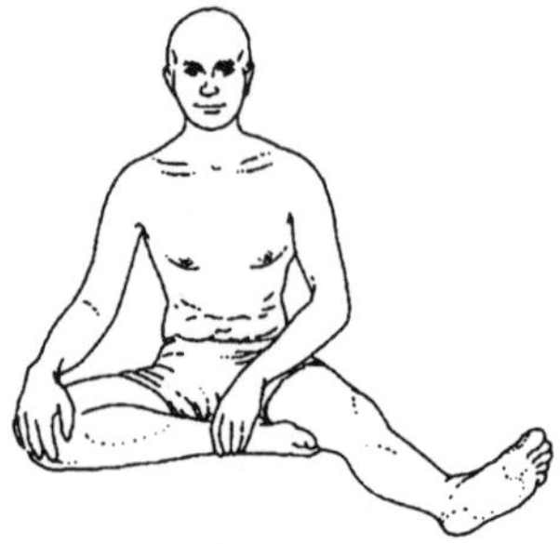

Bend your right leg at the knee. With both hands, place the right foot in such a way that the sole is touching the inside of the left thigh.

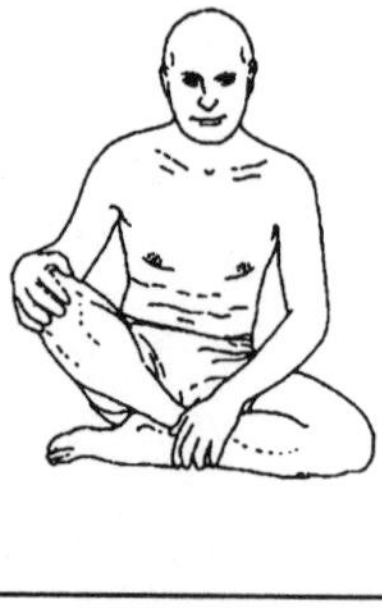

Now bend your left knee, holding the foot with your left hand, while the right hand keeps the right sole touching the left thigh.

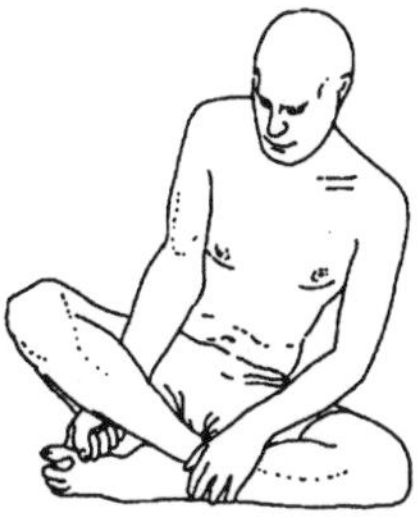

Slightly raise your right thigh and insert your right hand between your thigh and calf, and catch the big toe of the left foot with the index finger. Place the left foot in such a way that the left sole will be between the thigh and the calf.

Keep your body straight and hands in Jñâna Mudrâ. Keep the eyes closed or gaze at the tip of your nose.

Suggestions

1. Sit with your spine, neck, and head in a balanced condition.
2. Keep your soles touching the thighs.
3. The position can be reversed, if it is to be maintained for a long time.

Results

It has the advantages of a meditative pose, and is easy to maintain for a long time.

Discussion and References

Svastika means auspicious. Âsana means pose. Therefore, Svastikâsana means Auspicious Pose.

The legs cross each other above the ankles which indicates the mysterious Svastika.

This is a widely accepted pose which is mentioned in most of the traditional books on Yoga such as *H.P.* (I, 19), *Š.S.* (III, 115-117), and *S.S.P.* (II, 34)

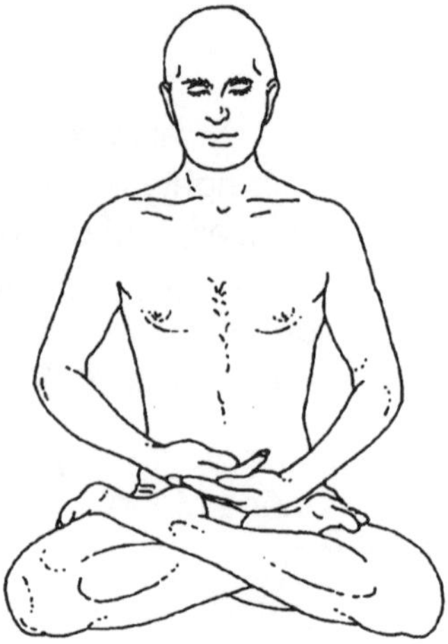

XXIII
PADMÂSANA
Lotus Pose

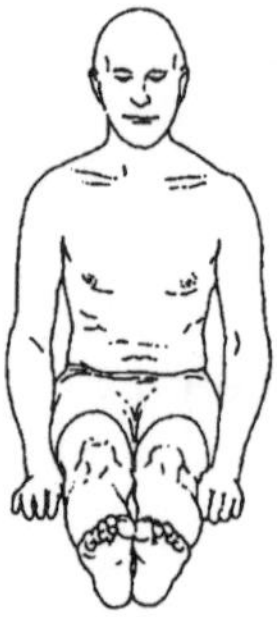

Technique

Sit with legs extended.

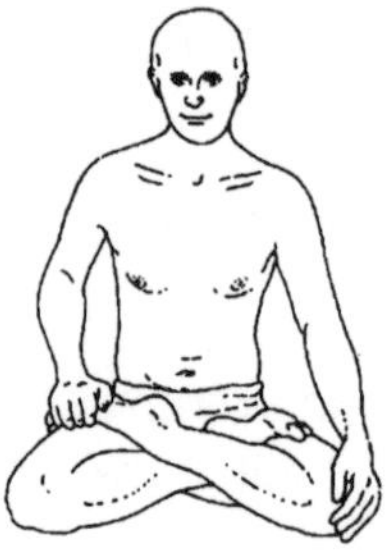

Place the right foot on the left thigh and the left foot on the right thigh, with soles turned upward.

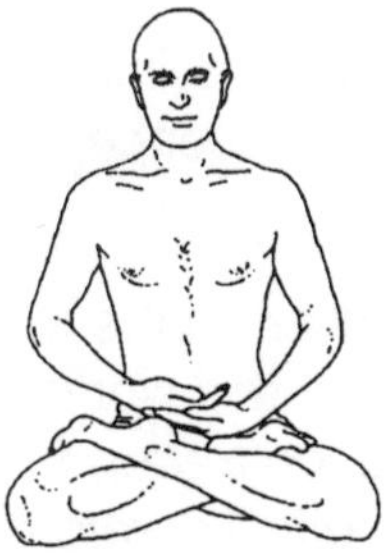

Place your left hand between the heels with palm upward, and your right hand on top of the left, with palm upward.

Sit erect with eyes closed or in a nasal gaze.

Suggestions

1. Maintain the spine, neck, and head in a balanced, erect condition.
2. Hold your knee as you are placing the foot on the thigh, in order to avoid overstrain.
3. Palms can also be placed on the knees in Jñâna Mudrâ, or left palm on top of right, depending on what is most comfortable for you at this stage.
4. If you find Padmâsana difficult, then first practice Vîrâsana (Hero Pose), with alternating legs. Learn to sit on the floor.

Results

It increases internal awareness by lowering reactivity to external stimuli. It provides a broader base to sit, giving greater stability. It tones the internal visceral organs and gives a richer blood supply to the pelvic region. It induces an attitude of calmness, if an aspirant follows a proper philosophy.

Discussion and References

Padma means lotus. Âsana means pose. Therefore, Padmâsana means Lotus Pose.

It resembles a lotus in physical appearance, if one imagines the soles and palms turned upward as leaves. But, in essence, the message is symbolic.

The lotus springs through mud and water and floats on the top untouched by both. In the same way, we are born of this world, yet it is possible to remain untouched by the world. Even a drop of water does not stay on a lotus leaf, but will slide off. Therefore, the lotus is considered a symbol of purity and untainted living.

Padmâsana is described as a most important pose. Practically all texts include Padmâsana as one of the sitting poses.

There are many variations of Padmâsana. In the first variation, the big toes are held by the hands with arms crossed behind the back. This is known as Baddha Padmâsana, or Bound Lotus. Other variations include changes in either placement of the hands or position of the lower extremities, or direction of the gaze. It can be done with Bandhas (locks) or without the Bandhas.

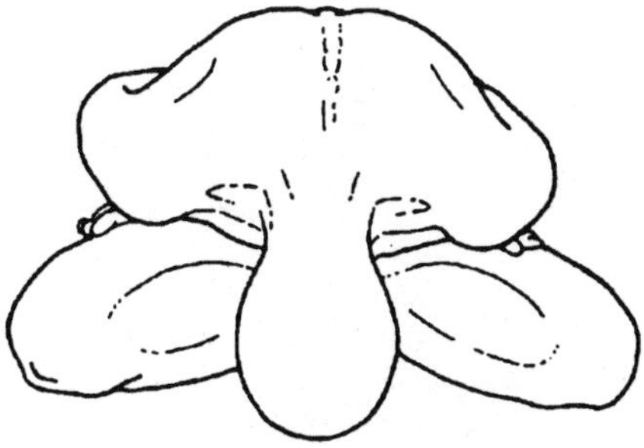

XXIV

YOGA MUDRÂ

Symbol of Yoga

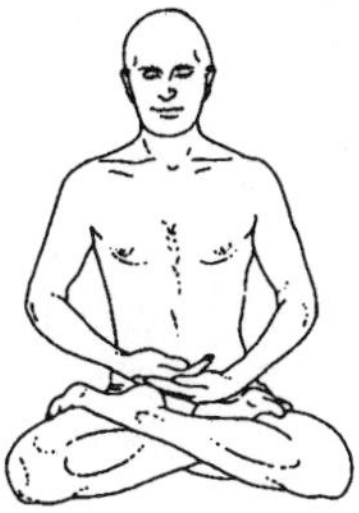

Technique

Sit in Padmâsana (Lotus Pose).

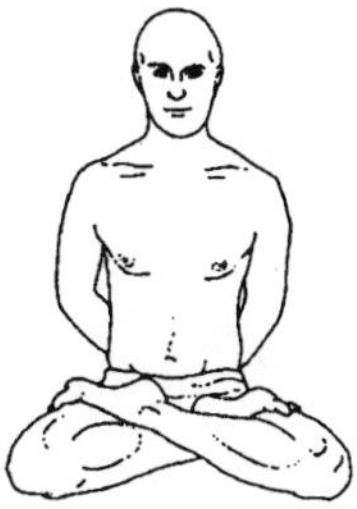

Bring your hands behind your back.

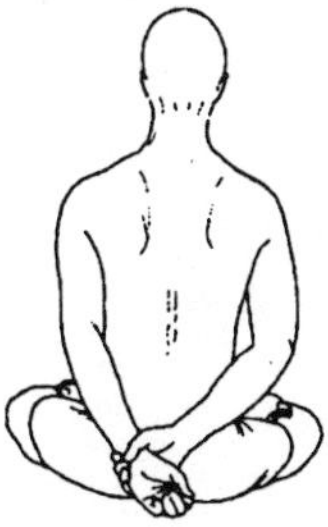

Grasp the left wrist in the right hand in a relaxed condition.

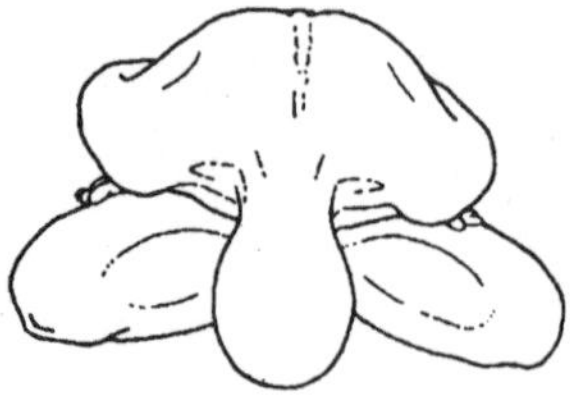

Bring your forehead to the ground by bending the trunk slowly and smoothly without jerks. Stay in the pose for some time.

Come back to the erect sitting position. Release your hands and legs and relax.

Suggestions

1. Avoid jerks of the spine.
2. If you cannot touch your forehead to the ground, make an attempt in a comfortable way, and maintain at that position.
3. Do not lift your buttocks in order to touch the floor.
4. Go through all the movements in a slow and smooth way.
5. Beginners and those who cannot assume the Lotus Pose, may use Vîrâsana (Hero Pose), Sukhâsana (Easy Pose), Vajrâsana (Pelvic Pose), or Svastikâsana (Auspicious Pose) described elsewhere in this book.

Results

It tones up the visceral organs and the nervous system. It reduces constipation, increases vitality, and helps in the arousal of Kuṇḍalinî (latent energies).

Discussion and References

Yoga means union. Mudrâ means symbol or attitude.

This practice indicates one of the important aspects of progress in

Yoga: surrender. Surrendering leads to receptivity and humility in learning. This type of surrender is not a blind slavery. It is an attitude.

This Mudrâ, practiced along with Âsanas, is not a Mudrâ in the strict technical sense of the term.

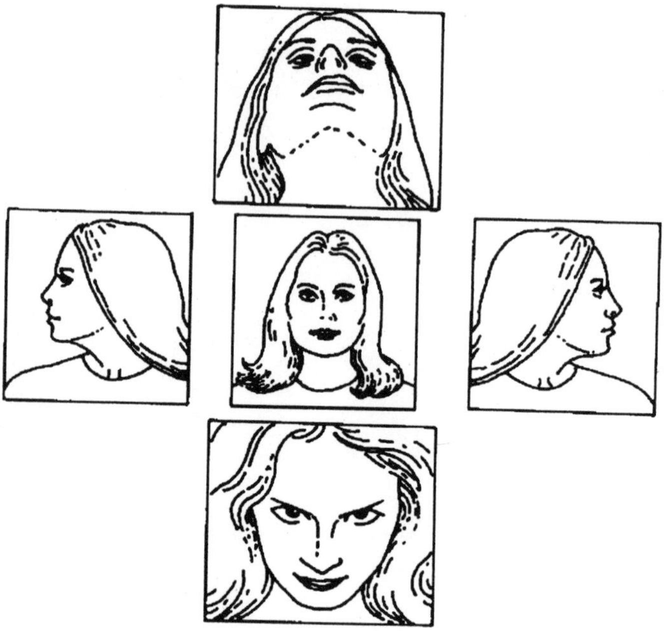

XXV

BRAHMA MUDRÂ

Symbol of Brahmâ

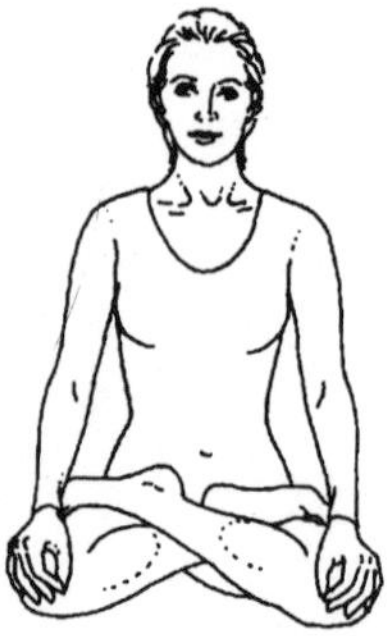

Technique

Sit in Padmâsana (Lotus Pose), or any other comfortable pose. Place your hands on the knees and look in front, in the line of your eyes.

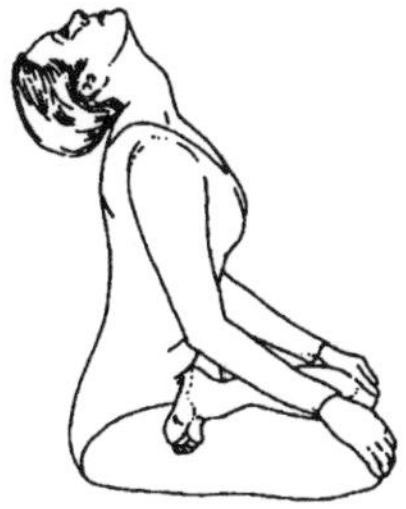

Stretch your head back and look at the tip of the nose. Maintain for a few seconds. Return to the original position.

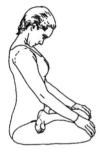

Place your chin in the jugular notch (depression of the throat), and look between the eyebrows. Hold for a few seconds. Return to the starting pose.

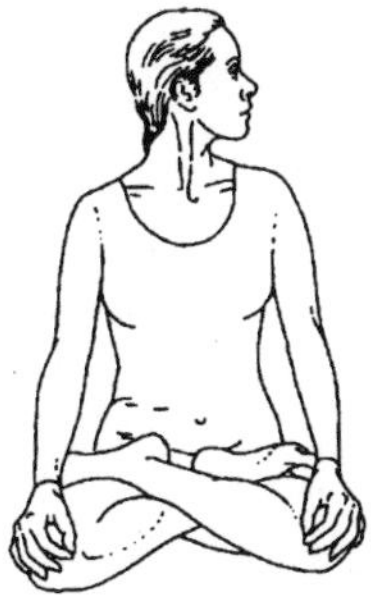

Now rotate your neck towards your left and look beyond your left shoulder. Hold for some time and return to the original position.

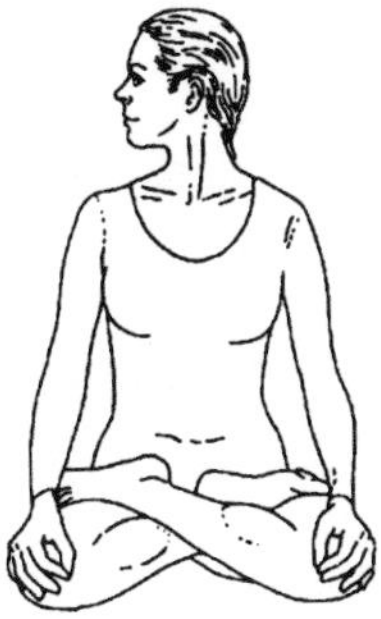

Rotate to the right and look beyond your right shoulder. Hold and come back to the original position.

Repeat the entire sequence two or three times.

Suggestions

1. Keep your mouth closed during this whole practice.
2. When stretching the neck back, keep the nasal gaze; similarly, when the chin is in the jugular notch, maintain the gaze between the eyebrows.
3. Do not move your shoulders.
4. If you feel uncomfortable with open eyes, first practice with closed eyes, imagining the tip of your nose and the space between your eyebrows.

Results

It is an excellent eye and neck exercise. It relieves tension in the neck, and strengthens the eye muscles.

It may also influence the thyroid and parathyroid glands.

Discussion and References

Of the traditional Hindu Trinity of Gods, Brahmâ is the Creator.

He is shown as having four heads in classical iconography; the heads being symbolic of the four Vedas. Therefore, this Mudrâ is named Brahma Mudrâ (*Yogic Therapy*, p. 62).

It seems that this practice influences Višuddha Cakra favorably; which according to tradition, leads to intuitive insight, enhances poetic talent, frees a person from depression, and gives longevity.

The mind becomes as clear as the sky — and therefore the name, Višuddha (pure as crystal), is given.

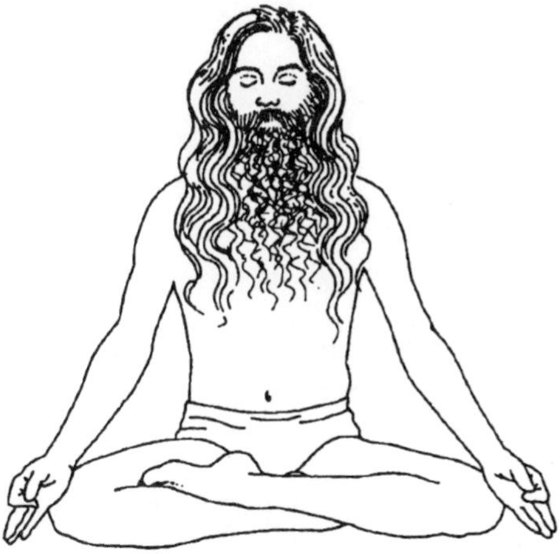

XXVI
UJJÂYÎ
Breathing with Sound (First Stage)

Technique

Sit in any comfortable meditative pose.

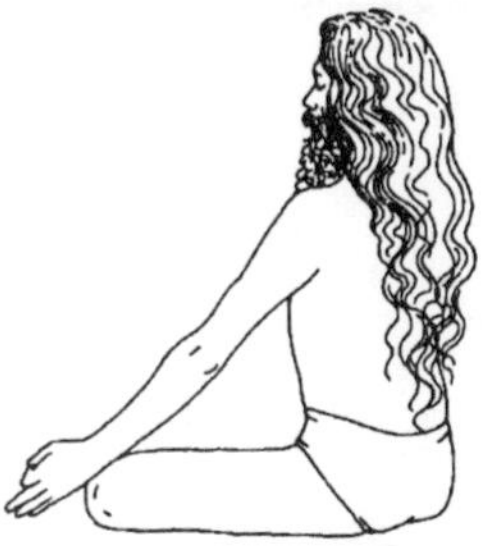

Raise the chest first while inhaling, then imagine the expansion of the rib cage, and then the abdomen. Keep the abdomen slightly contracted.

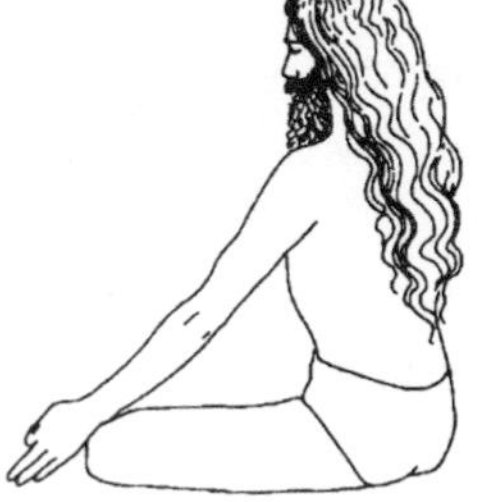

Then follow the reverse order in exhalation: contract the abdomen, rib cage, and finally chest, but without too much movement of the chest.

Take the breath in with a partial closure of the glottis, as a person does in snoring, but in a smooth, rhythmic, controlled way.

Then exhale with the sound.

Learn from a Yoga teacher how to produce the proper sound.

You can also try this method to produce the proper sound: exhale through your mouth with a "ha" sound, then do the same with your mouth closed.

After mastering the exhaling phase, try inhaling with sound.

According to tradition, Pûraka (inhaling) through both nostrils, Kumbhaka (retention), and Recaka (exhaling) through the left nostril is prescribed (*H.P.* II, 51-53).

It is suggested that beginners only practice the inhaling and exhaling phases, using both nostrils, with a natural pause between the two.

Close your eyes and attend to the sound you produce.

Repeat ten times or so, increasing gradually only if you are comfortable.

Suggestions

1. Do not bother, at the beginning stage, with the ratio of inhalation and exhalation, as is often mentioned in the Yogic literature.
2. Learn to breathe with sound, rhythmically and smoothly, with both nostrils.
3. Slowly, gradually, increase the duration.
4. If a nostril is so clogged that you cannot breathe properly, learn nasal cleansing practices from your teacher.

5. Exhale first before you start Pûraka.
6. Start with ten cycles; increase gradually under the supervision of a teacher.

Results

It helps to overcome tension and to vitalize the body in general, and the nervous system in particular. It relieves depression and may induce deeper states of consciousness. If properly guided, it is very helpful.

Discussion and References

The meaning of the word Ujjâyî is "that which leads to success" (*Prâṇâyâma*, p.52). The traditional method for inhaling through both nostrils and exhaling through the left seems to practically double the duration of exhalation.

Inhalation in Yogic breathing is done in a particular manner and therefore, in Yogic terminology, the word Pûraka is used, which is a different word than the word for normal inhalation, Švâsa. So is the case with Yogic exhalation, or Recaka, as differentiated from normal exhalation, Prašvâsa.

Yogic retention is known as Kumbhaka, which is different than normal retention, or holding the breath.

These terms, Pûraka, Kumbhaka, and Recaka are used for various Prâṇâyâma, or breath control techniques; i.e., the style of inhalation and exhalation differs among the techniques (*H.P.* II, 46- 48).

Prâṇâyâma occupies a special place in Yogic literature.

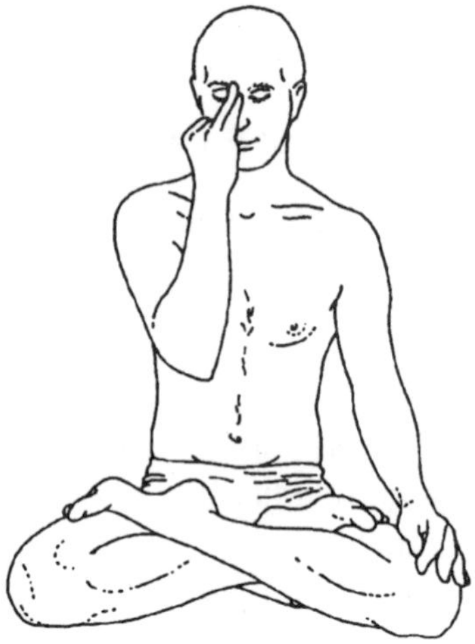

XXVII

UJJÂYÎ +

Breathing with Sound (Second Stage)

Technique

Sit in any comfortable meditative pose.

Take breath in through both nostrils with partial closure of the glottis, in a controlled way, as in the first stage.

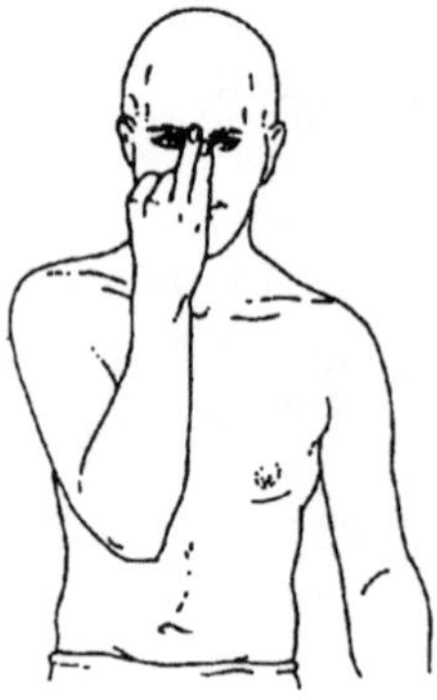

Place your thumb at the right nostril, keeping the ring finger and little finger at the bridge of the nose, preferably with the ring finger touching the point between the eyebrows.

Exhale through the left nostril, again with partial closure of the glottis, slowly and rhythmically.

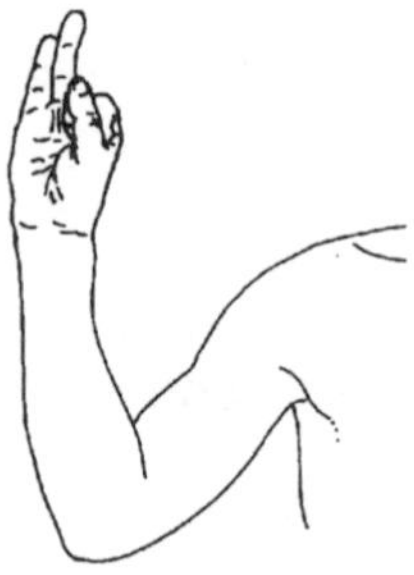

Suggestions

1. Start this practice only after mastering the first stage.
2. Increase the number of cycles gradually and cautiously.
3. Avoid forceful and sharp exhalation.
4. While switching from Pûraka (inhalation) to Recaka (exhalation), let it be smooth, like a wave.
5. Avoid unnecessary movements of the body.
6. Keep your face calm and pleasant.

Results

The results are the same as for the first stage, but it gives you better control in regulating your breath.

Discussion and References

According to tradition, Pûraka, Kumbhaka, and Recaka are prescribed for the general practice of Prâṇâyâma with a ratio of 1:4:2.

That is, if Pûraka is eight counts, Kumbhaka will be thirty-two counts, and Recaka will be sixteen counts. This practice seems to provide Pûraka and Recaka ratios of 1:2 without much effort.

For example, if you inhale through both nostrils in a specified period of time, logically it will take double the time to exhale through one nostril, using the same force. Therefore, Ujjâyî is considered a preliminary practice in learning to regulate the Pûraka and Recaka phases.

Ujjâyî is the effortful lifting (Âkṛṣya) of the breath from the navel.

8 Progressive Practice Plans

Each of the following 2-page practice plans provides a series of postures with breathing and relaxation techniques.

Stay on each level until you are thoroughly comfortable with the suggested repetitions and timing.

There is no hurry to move on. The process is more important than the final posture. Slow and steady wins the race!

Read the Helpful Hints at the front of this book before you begin, and refer to the posture's detailed description.

Do not compete with others, with the clock, or even with yourself. You are unique!

Note: The author cannot take responsibility for the improper use of these practices.

ŠAVÂSANA (Corpse Pose)	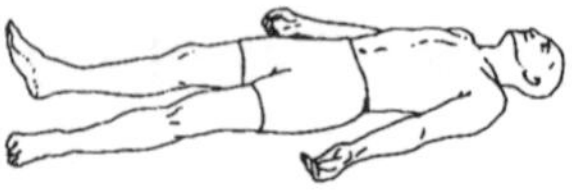	3 min.	p. 21
BHUJAṄGÂSANA (Cobra Pose)	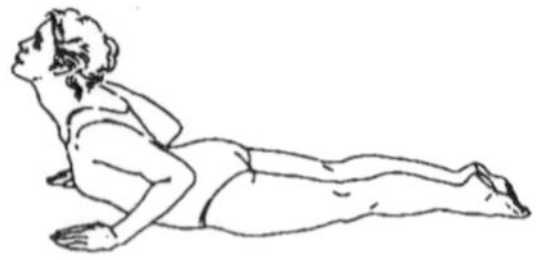	3 rounds (10 sec. each)	p. 23
ARDHA- ŠALABHÂSANA (Half-Locust Pose)	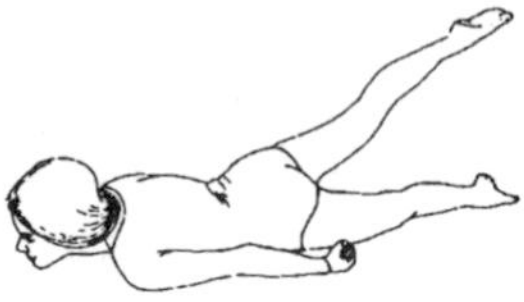	3 rounds (10 sec. each side)	p. 26
MAKARÂSANA (Crocodile Pose)	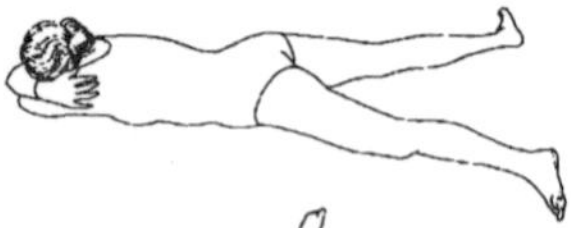	2 minutes	p. 32
ARDHA-HALÂSANA (Half-Plow Pose) first stage	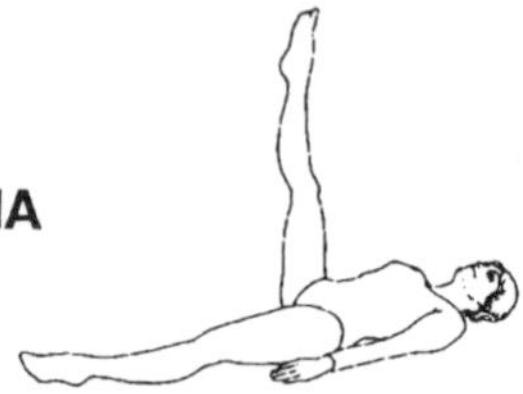	3 rounds (10 sec. each side)	p. 34
DAṆḌÂSANA (Stick Pose)	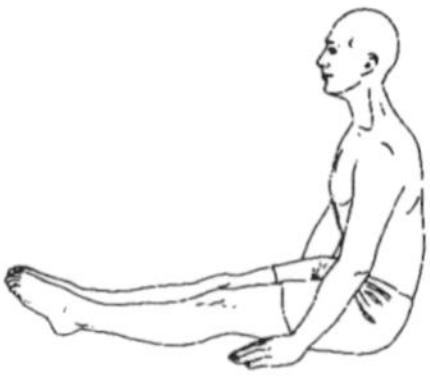	3 rounds (30 sec. each)	p. 41
VAKRÂSANA (Twist Pose)	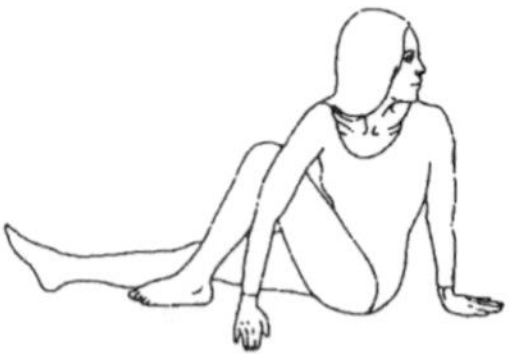	3 rounds (15 sec. each side)	p. 43

STAMBHÂSANA (Pillar Pose)	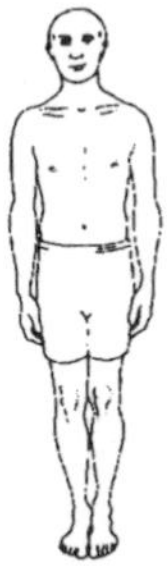	1 min.	p. 52
CAKRÂSANA (Side-Bending Pose)	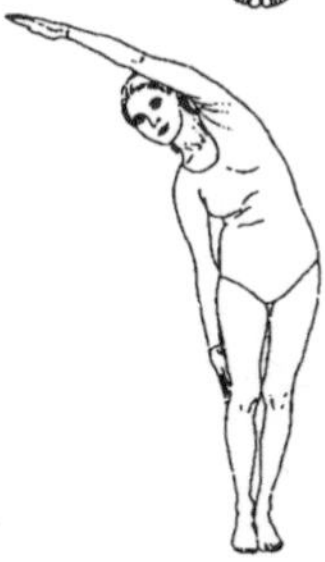	3 rounds (10 sec. each side)	p. 54
SUKHÂSANA (Easy Pose)	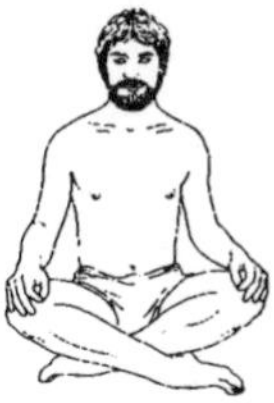	1 min.	p. 68
YOGA MUDRÂ (Symbol of Yoga)	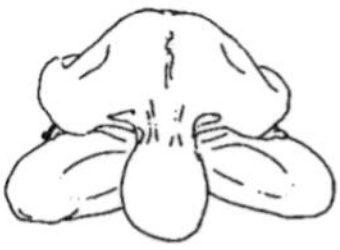	3 rounds (30 sec. each)	p. 79
UJJÂYÎ (Breathing with Sound) first stage	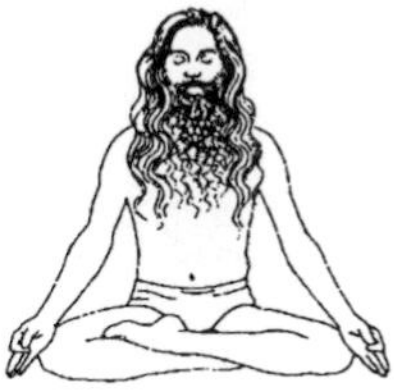	10 rounds	p. 85
ŠAVÂSANA (Corpse Pose)	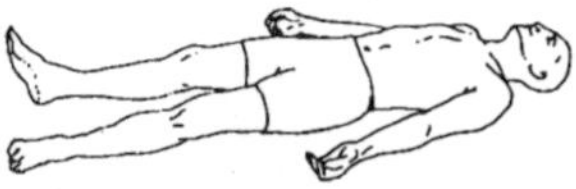	3 min.	p. 21

BHUJAṄGÂSANA (Cobra Pose)	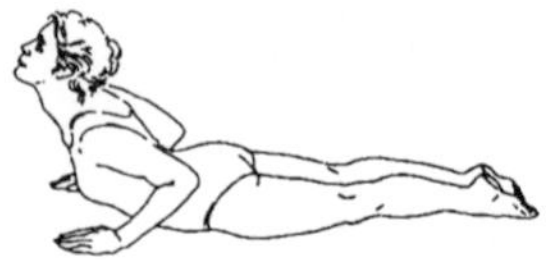	3 rounds (10 sec. each)	p. 23
ARDHA-ŠALABHÂSANA (Half-Locust Pose)	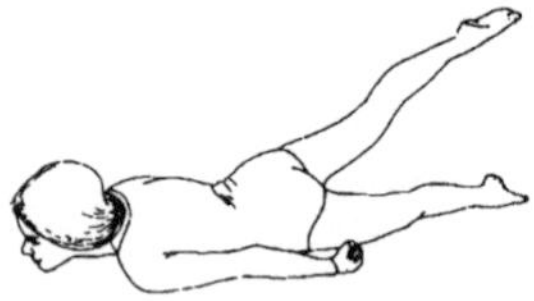	3 rounds (10 sec. each side)	p. 26
DHANURÂSANA (Bow Pose)	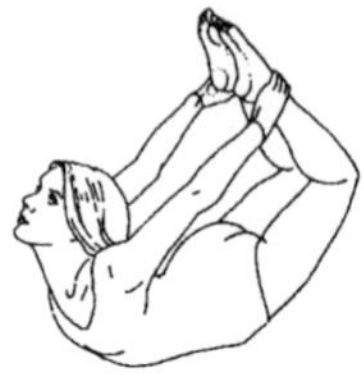	3 rounds (10 sec. each)	p. 30
MAKARÂSANA (Crocodile Pose)	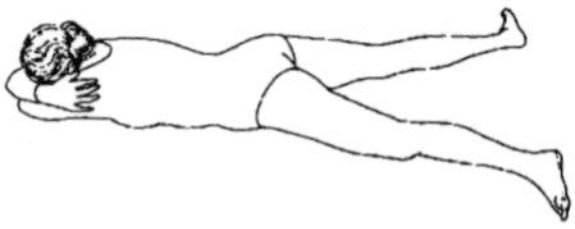	2 minutes	p. 32
ARDHA-HALÂSANA (Half-Plow Pose) first stage	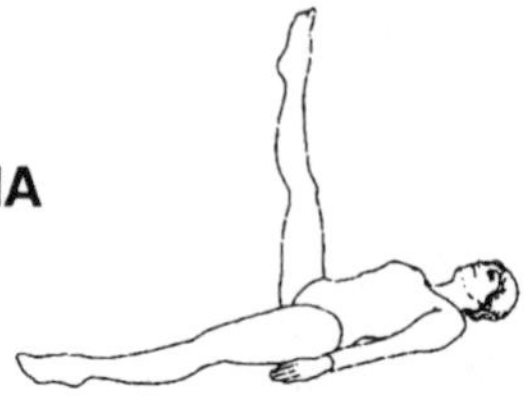	3 rounds (10 sec. each side)	p. 34
ARDHA-HALÂSANA (Half-Plow Pose) second stage	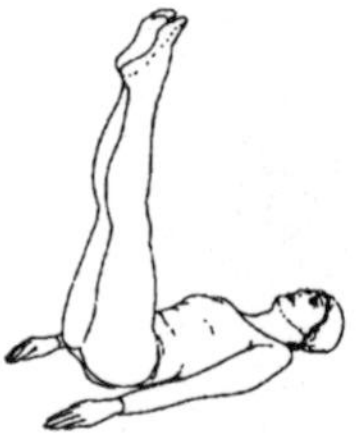	3 rounds (10 sec. each)	p. 36
PAŠCIMATÂNÂSANA (Posterior Stretch Pose)	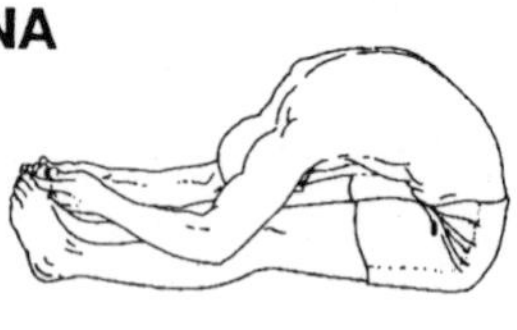	2 rounds (15 sec. each)	p. 49

VAKRÂSANA (Twist Pose)	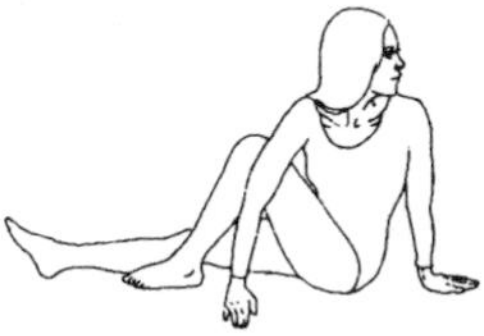	3 rounds (15 sec. each side)	p. 43
CAKRÂSANA (Side-Bending Pose)	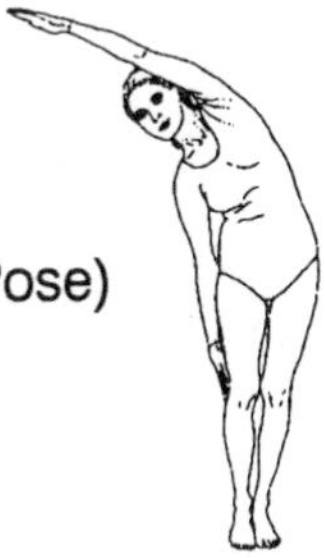	3 rounds (10 sec. each side)	p. 54
VṚKṢÂSANA (Tree Pose)	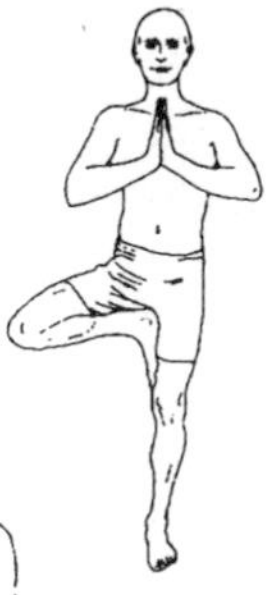	3 rounds (10 sec. each side)	p. 57
VAJRÂSANA (Pelvic Pose)	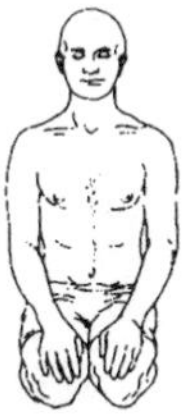	1 minute	p. 65
YOGA MUDRÂ (Symbol of Yoga)	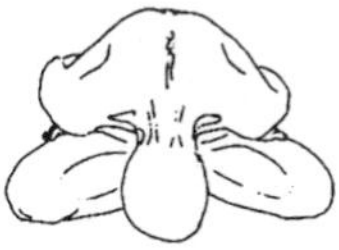	3 rounds (30 sec. each)	p. 79
UJJÂYÎ (Breathing with Sound) first stage	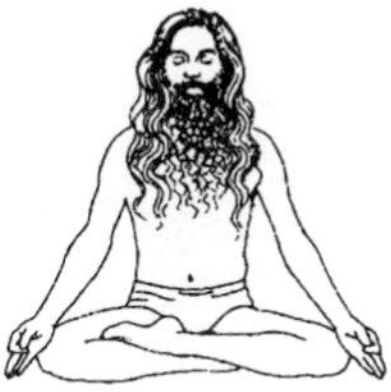	10 rounds	p. 85
ŠAVÂSANA (Corpse Pose)	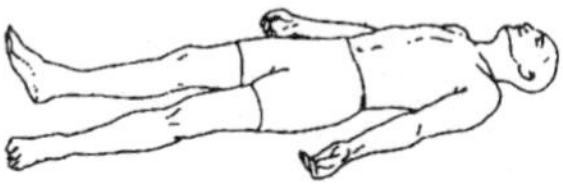	3 min.	p. 21

BHUJAṄGÂSANA (Cobra Pose)	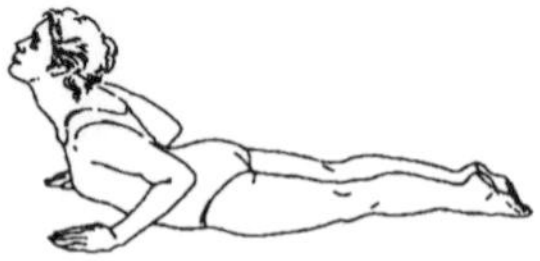	3 rounds (10 sec. each)	p. 23
ŠALABHÂSANA (Locust Pose)	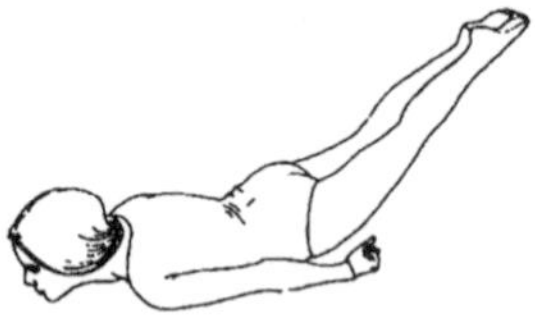	3 rounds (10 sec. each)	p. 28
DHANURÂSANA (Bow Pose)	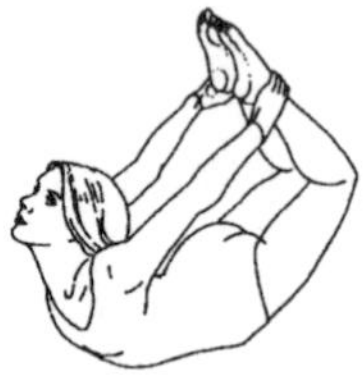	3 rounds (10 sec. each)	p. 30
MAKARÂSANA (Crocodile Pose)	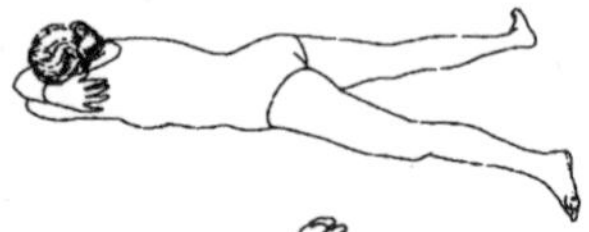	2 minutes	p. 32
ARDHA-HALÂSANA (Half-Plow Pose) second stage	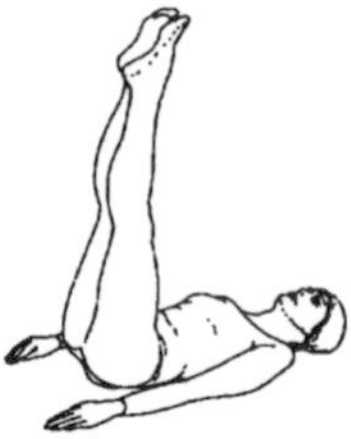	3 rounds (10 sec. each)	p. 36
PAŠCIMATÂNÂSANA (Posterior Stretch Pose)	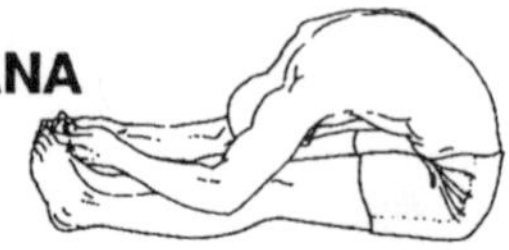	2 rounds (30 sec. each)	p. 49
VAKRÂSANA (Twist Pose)	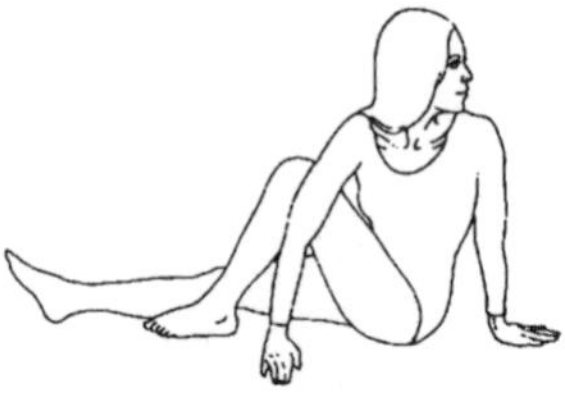	3 rounds (30 sec. each side)	p. 43

CAKRÂSANA (Side-Bending Pose)	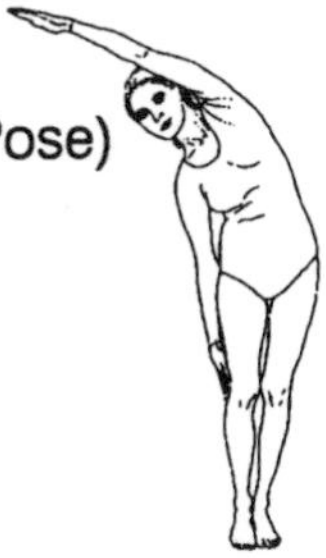	3 rounds (10 sec. each side)	p. 54
VṚKṢÂSANA (Tree Pose)	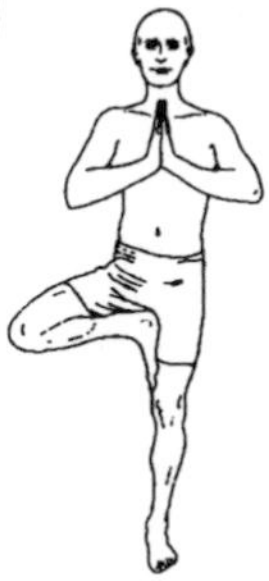	3 rounds (15 sec. each side)	p. 57
SAṄKAṬÂSANA (Difficult Pose)	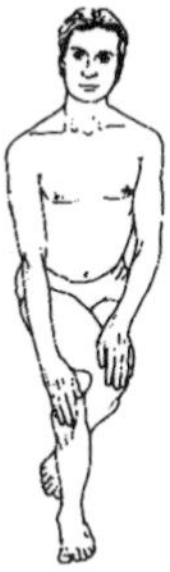	3 rounds (10 sec. each side)	p. 60
VÎRÂSANA (Hero Pose)	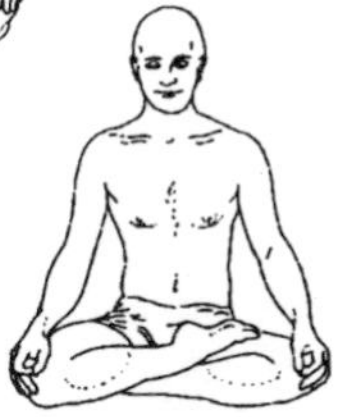	1 minute	p. 71
BRAHMA MUDRÂ (Symbol of Brahmâ)	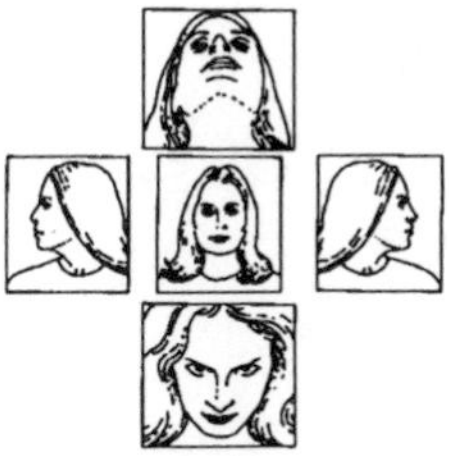	2 rounds (3 sec. each posi- tion)	p. 82
UJJÂYÎ (Breathing with Sound) first stage	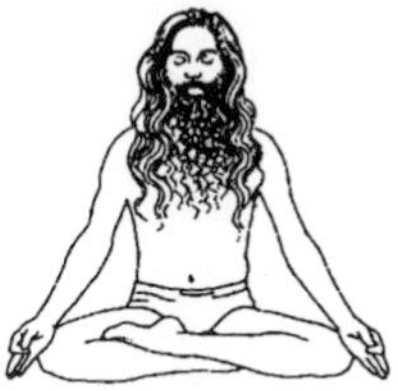	10 rounds	p. 85
ŠAVÂSANA (Corpse Pose)	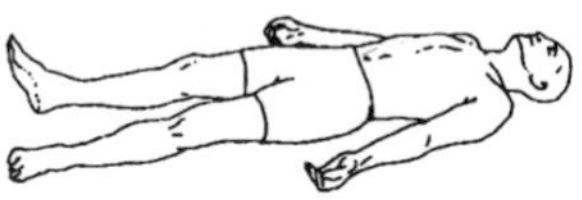	3 min.	p. 21

BHUJAṄGÂSANA (Cobra Pose)	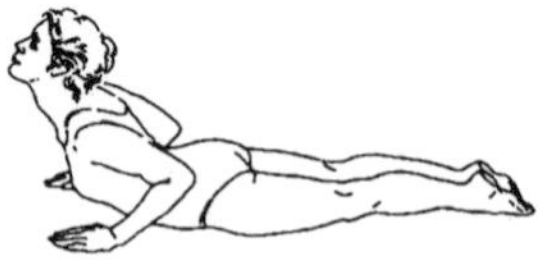	3 rounds (10 sec. each)	p. 23
ŠALABHÂSANA (Locust Pose)	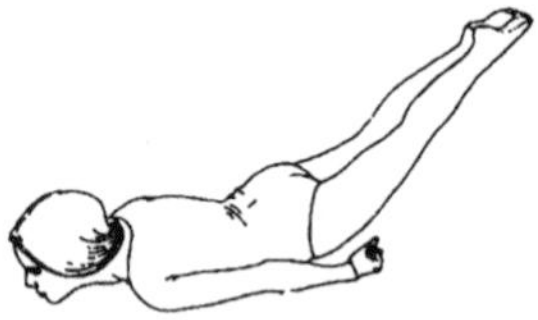	3 rounds (10 sec. each)	p. 28
DHANURÂSANA (Bow Pose)	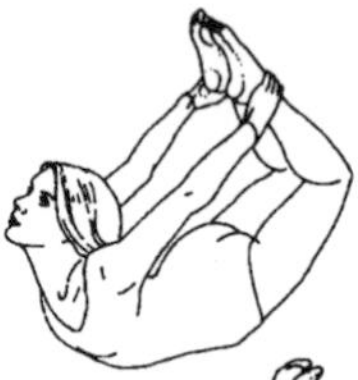	3 rounds (10 sec. each)	p. 30
ARDHA-HALÂSANA (Half-Plow Pose) second stage	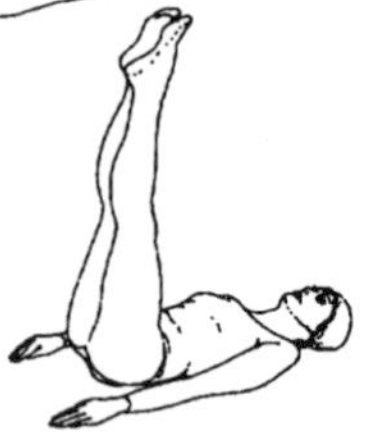	3 rounds (15 sec. each)	p. 36
HALÂSANA (Plow Pose)	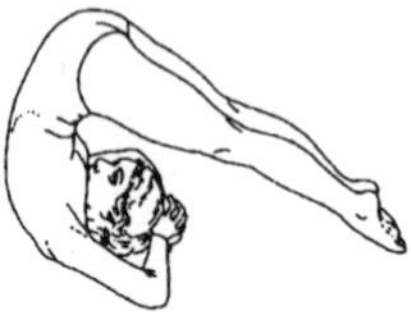	1 round (1 minute)	p. 38
PAŠCIMATÂNÂSANA (Posterior Stretch Pose)	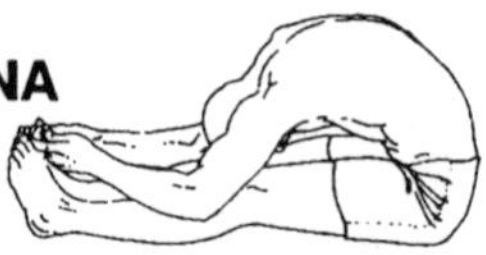	1 round (1 minute)	p. 49
VAKRÂSANA (Twist Pose)	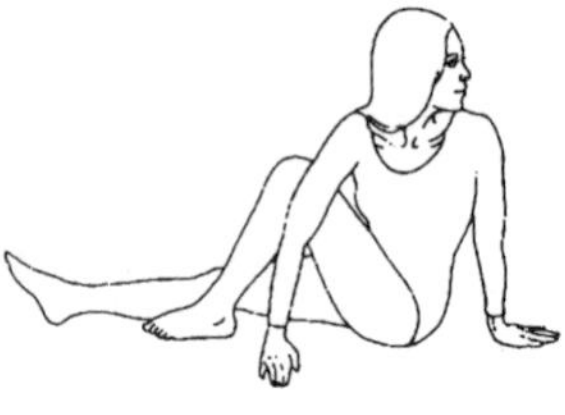	3 rounds (30 sec. each side)	p. 43

CAKRÂSANA (Side-Bending Pose)	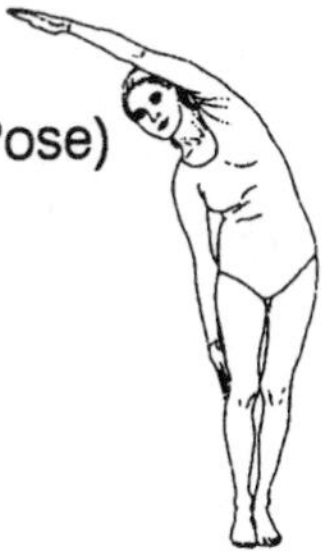	3 rounds (10 sec. each side)	p. 54
VṚKṢÂSANA (Tree Pose)	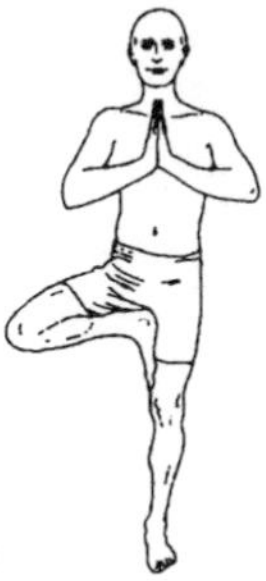	3 rounds (15 sec. each side)	p. 57
SAṄKAṬÂSANA (Difficult Pose)	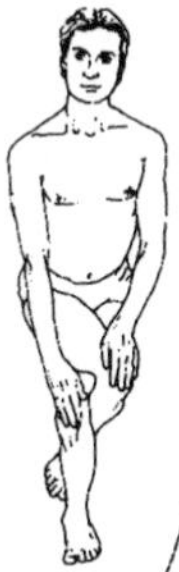	3 rounds (10 sec. each side)	p. 60
PADMÂSANA (Lotus Pose)	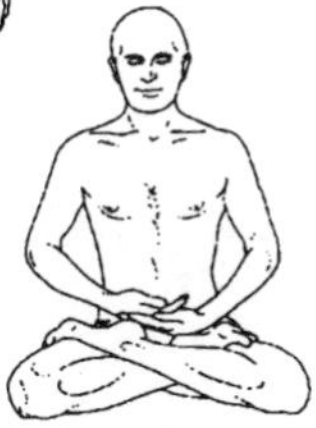	1 minute	p. 76
BRAHMA MUDRÂ (Symbol of Brahmâ)	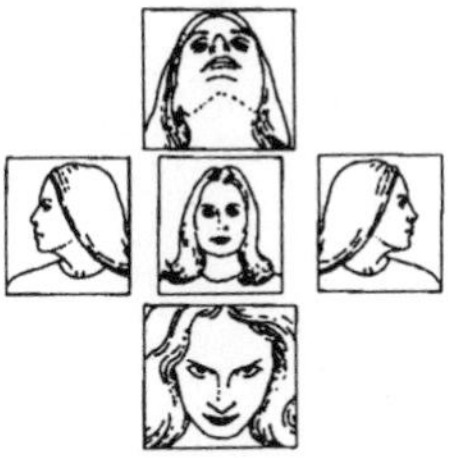	2 rounds (3 sec. each position)	p. 82
UJJÂYÎ (Breathing with Sound) first stage	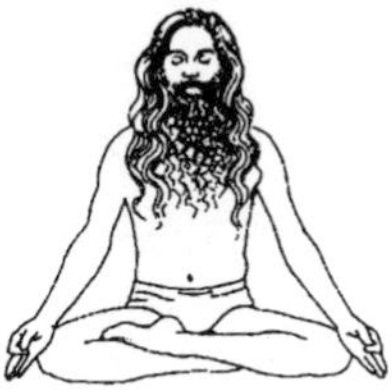	10 rounds	p. 85
ŠAVÂSANA (Corpse Pose)	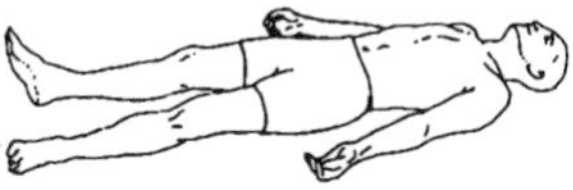	3 min.	p. 21

BHUJAṄGÂSANA (Cobra Pose)	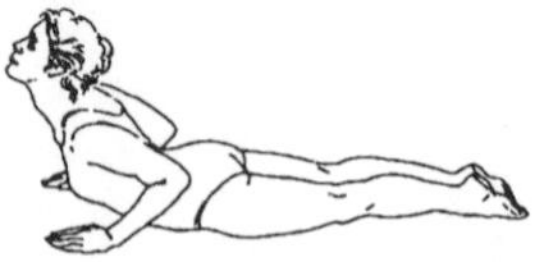	3 rounds (10 sec. each)	p. 23
ŠALABHÂSANA (Locust Pose)	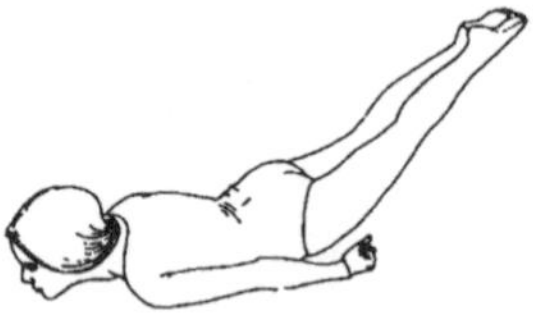	3 rounds (10 sec. each)	p. 28
DHANURÂSANA (Bow Pose)	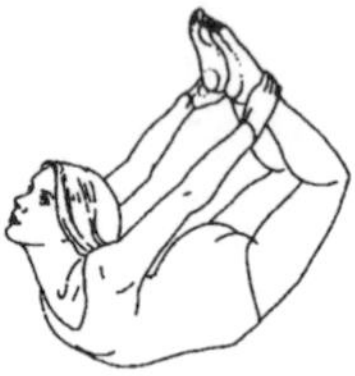	3 rounds (10 sec. each)	p. 30
MAKARÂSANA (Crocodile Pose)	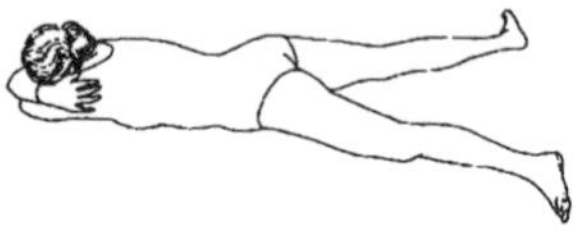	2 minutes	p. 32
HALÂSANA (Plow Pose)	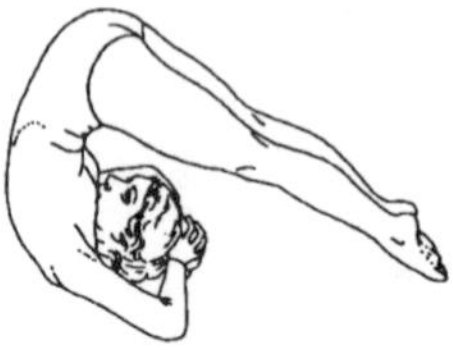	1 round (1 minute)	p. 38
ARDHA-MATSYENDRÂSANA (Half-Matsyendra Pose)	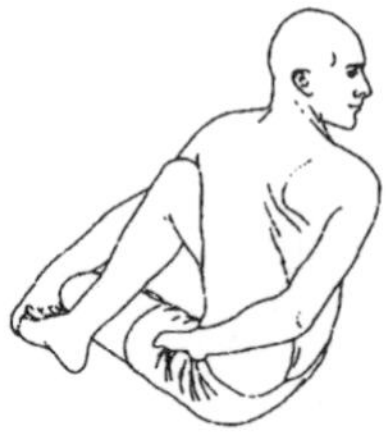	3 rounds (10 sec. each side)	p. 46
PAŠCIMATÂNÂSANA (Posterior Stretch Pose)	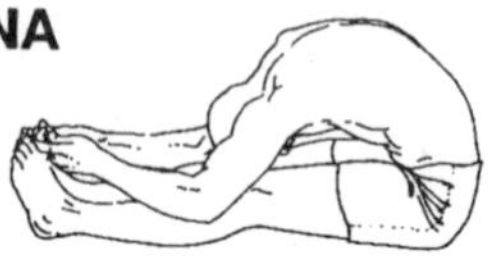	1 round (1 minute)	p. 49

CAKRÂSANA (Side-Bending Pose)	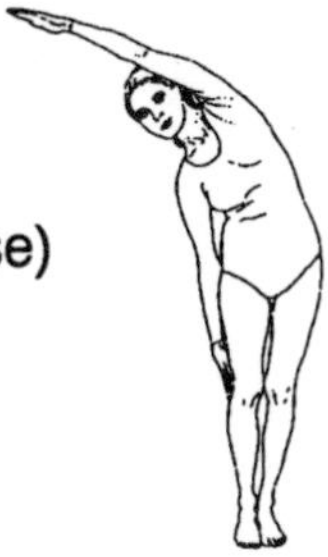	2 rounds (15 sec. each side)	p. 54
VṚKṢÂSANA (Tree Pose)	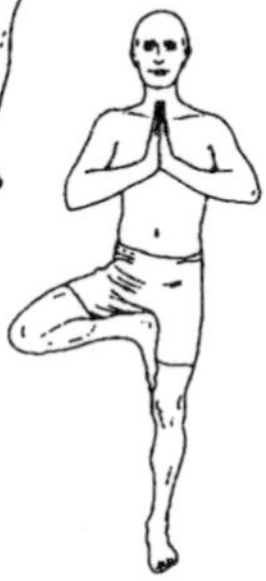	3 rounds (15 sec. each side)	p. 57
SAṄKAṬÂSANA (Difficult Pose)	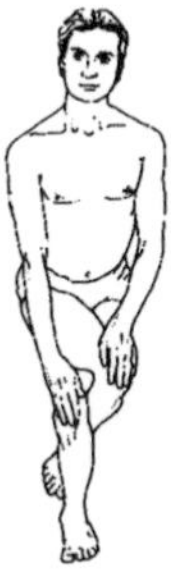	2 rounds (15 sec. each side)	p. 60
SVASTIKÂSANA (Auspicious Pose)	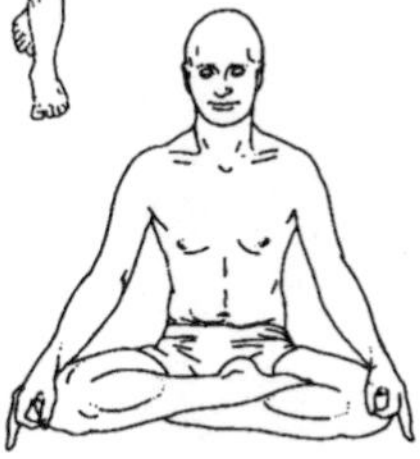	1 minute	p. 74
YOGA MUDRÂ (Symbol of Yoga)	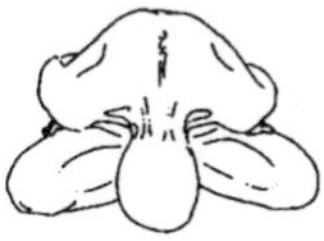	2 rounds (1 min. each)	p. 79
UJJÂYÎ (Breathing with Sound) second stage	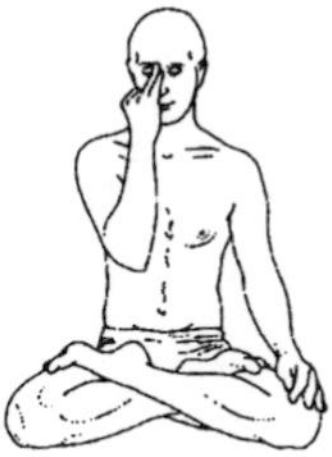	10 rounds	p. 85
ŠAVÂSANA (Corpse Pose)	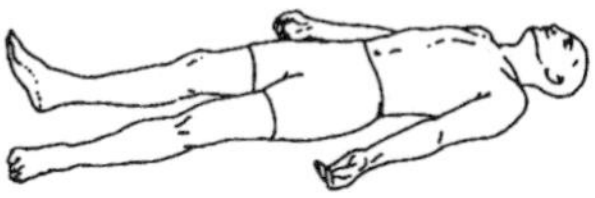	5 min.	p. 21

BHUJAṄGÂSANA
(Cobra Pose)

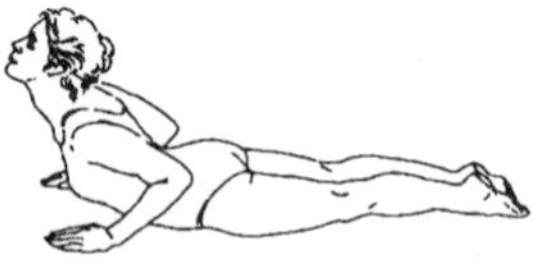

3 rounds (10 sec. each) p. 23

ŠALABHÂSANA
(Locust Pose)

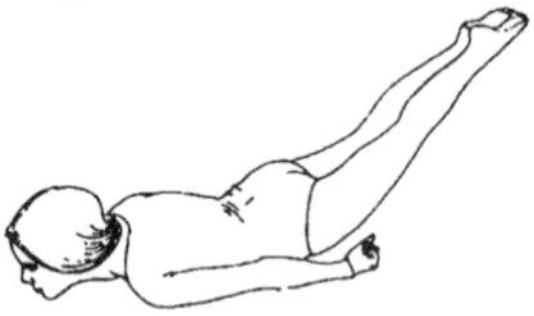

3 rounds (10 sec. each) p. 28

DHANURÂSANA
(Bow Pose)

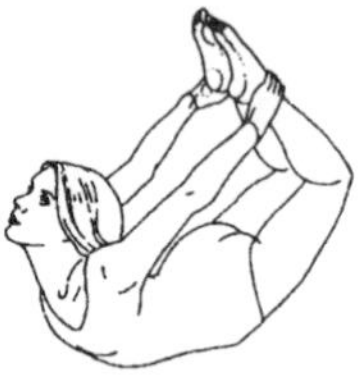

3 rounds (10 sec. each) p. 30

HALÂSANA
(Plow Pose)

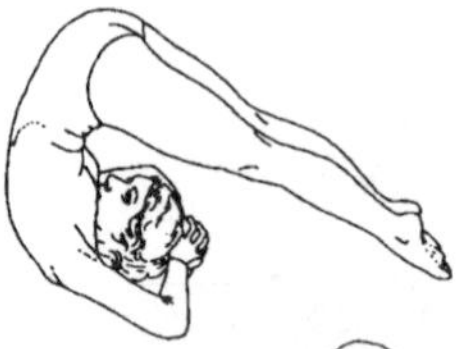

1 round (2 minutes) p. 38

ARDHA-MATSYENDRÂSANA
(Half-Matsyendra Pose)

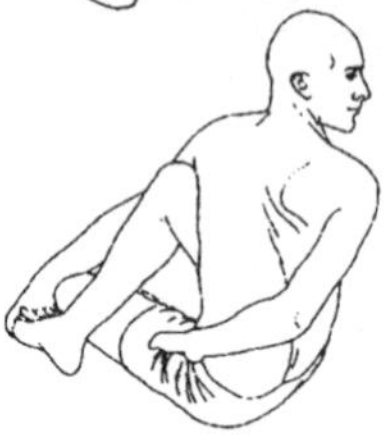

2 rounds (20 sec. each side) p. 46

PAŠCIMATÂNÂSANA
(Posterior Stretch Pose)

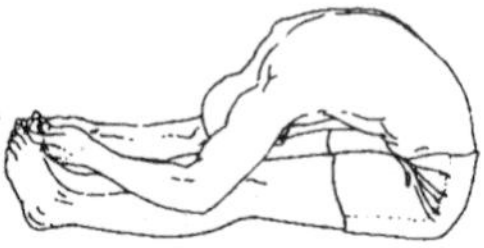

1 round (1 minute) p. 49

VṚKṢÂSANA
(Tree Pose)

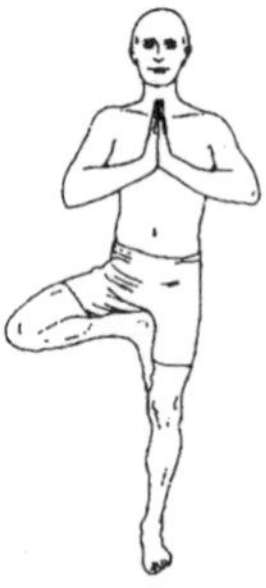

3 rounds (15 sec. each side) p. 57

SAṄKAṬÂSANA (Difficult Pose)	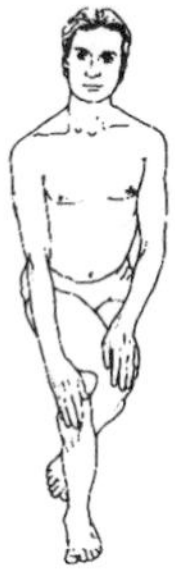	2 rounds (15 sec. each side)	p. 60
PÂDAHASTÂSANA (Hand-to-Foot Pose)	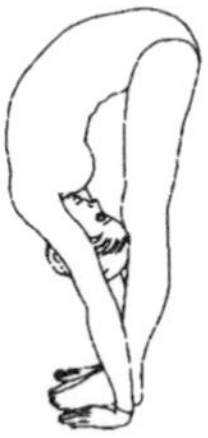	2 rounds (10 sec. each)	p. 63
SVASTIKÂSANA (Auspicious Pose)	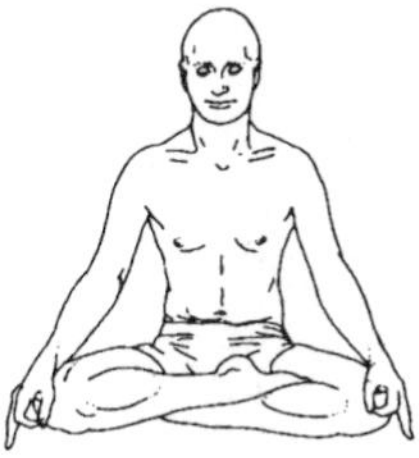	1 minute	p. 74
BRAHMA MUDRÂ (Symbol of Brahmâ)	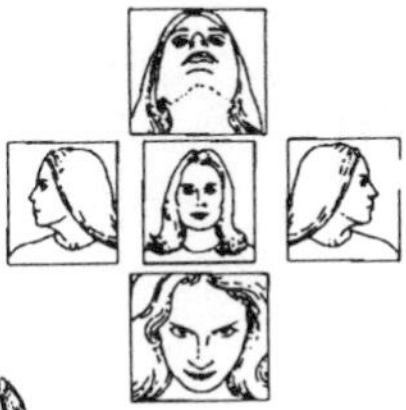	3 rounds (3 sec. each position)	p. 82
UJJÂYÎ (Breathing with Sound) first stage	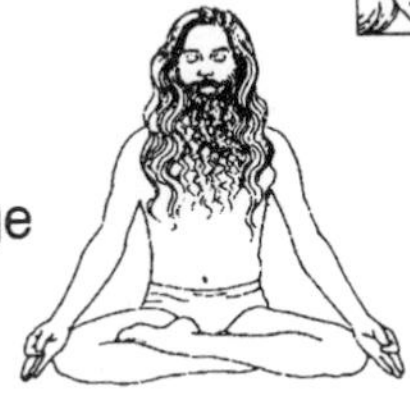	10 rounds	p. 85
UJJÂYÎ (Breathing with Sound) second stage	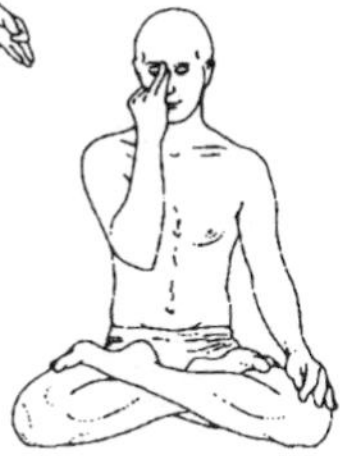	5 rounds	p. 88
ŠAVÂSANA (Corpse Pose)	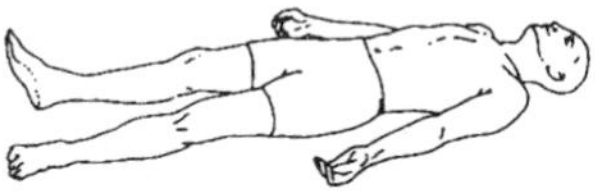	5 min.	p. 21

BHUJAṄGÂSANA (Cobra Pose)	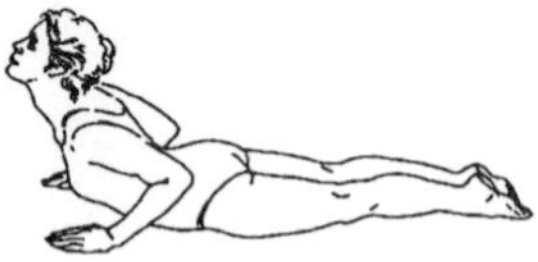	4 rounds (10 sec. each)	p. 23
ŠALABHÂSANA (Locust Pose)	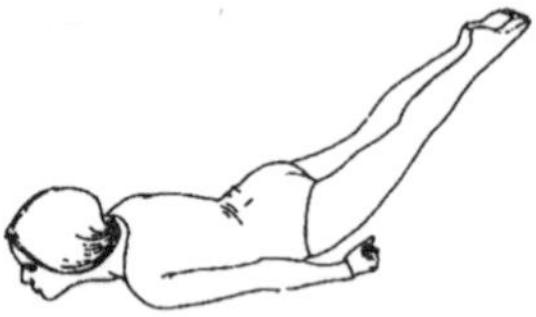	4 rounds (10 sec. each)	p. 28
DHANURÂSANA (Bow Pose)	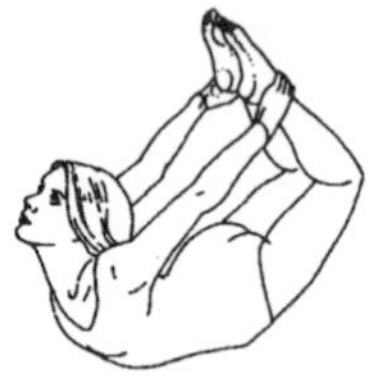	4 rounds (10 sec. each)	p. 30
HALÂSANA (Plow Pose)	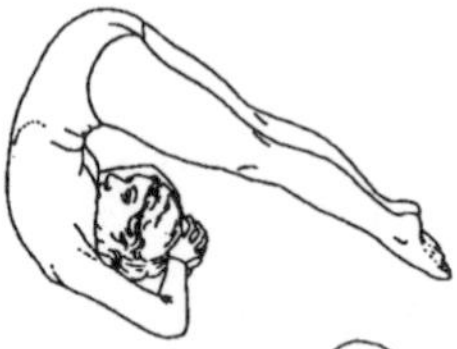	1 round (2 minutes)	p. 38
ARDHA-MATSYENDRÂSANA (Half-Matsyendra Pose)	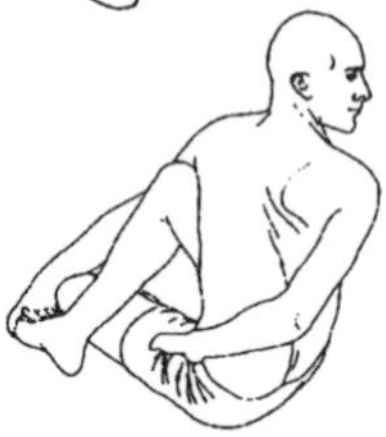	2 rounds (30 sec. each side)	p. 46
PAŠCIMATÂNÂSANA (Posterior Stretch Pose)	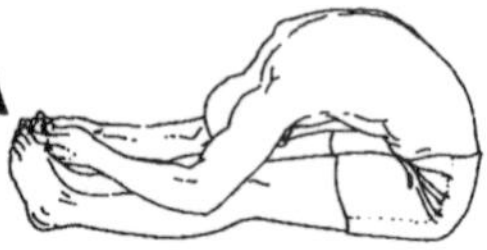	1 round (1 minute)	p. 49
VṚKṢÂSANA (Tree Pose)	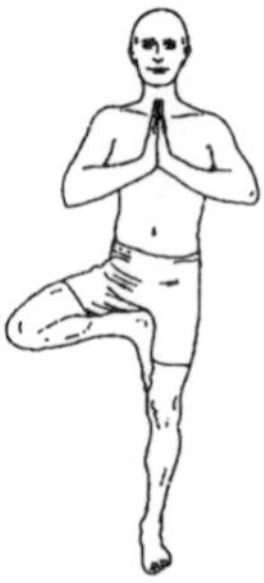	2 rounds (45 sec. each side)	p. 57

SAṄKAṬÂSANA (Difficult Pose)	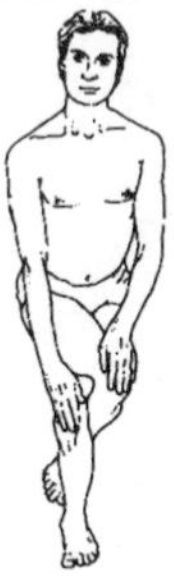	2 rounds (15 sec. each side)	p. 60
PÂDAHASTÂSANA (Hand-to-Foot Pose)	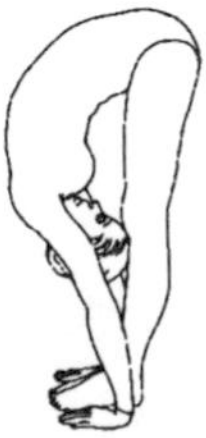	2 rounds (10 sec. each)	p. 63
BRAHMA MUDRÂ (Symbol of Brahmâ)	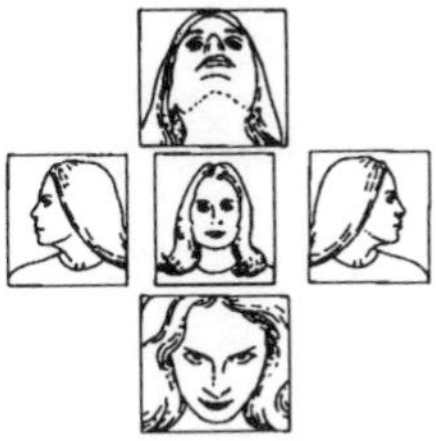	2 rounds (5 sec. each position)	p. 82
YOGA MUDRÂ (Symbol of Yoga)	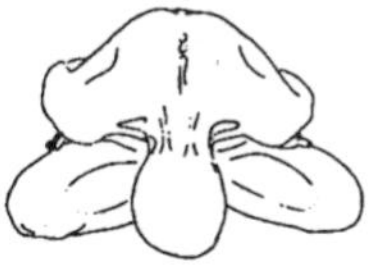	1 round (2 minutes)	p. 79
UJJÂYÎ (Breathing with Sound) first stage	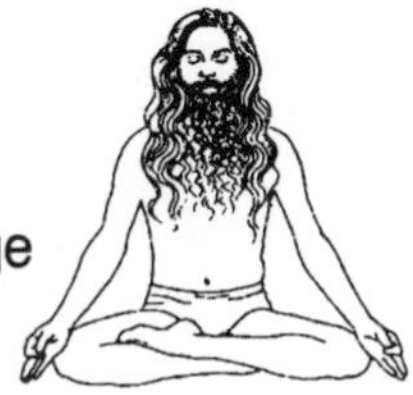	10 rounds	p. 85
UJJÂYÎ (Breathing with Sound) second stage	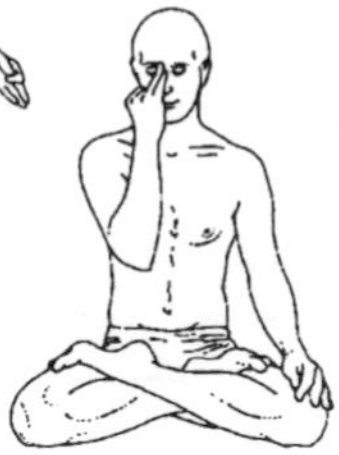	5 rounds	p. 88
ŠAVÂSANA (Corpse Pose)	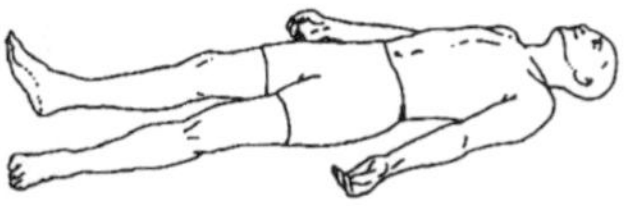	5 min.	p. 21

BHUJAṄGÂSANA (Cobra Pose)	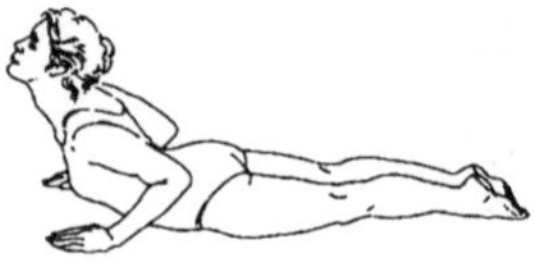	4 rounds (10 sec. each)	p. 23
ŠALABHÂSANA (Locust Pose)	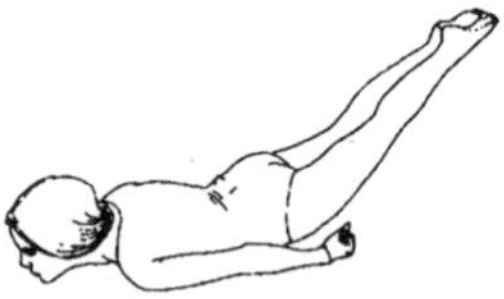	4 rounds (10 sec. each)	p. 28
DHANURÂSANA (Bow Pose)	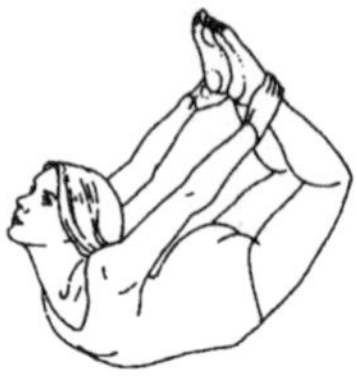	4 rounds (10 sec. each)	p. 30
HALÂSANA (Plow Pose)	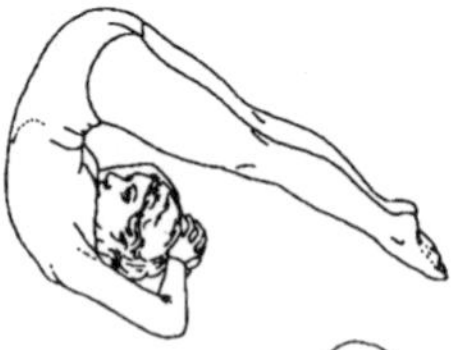	1 round (2 minutes)	p. 38
ARDHA-MATSYENDRÂSANA (Half-Matsyendra Pose)	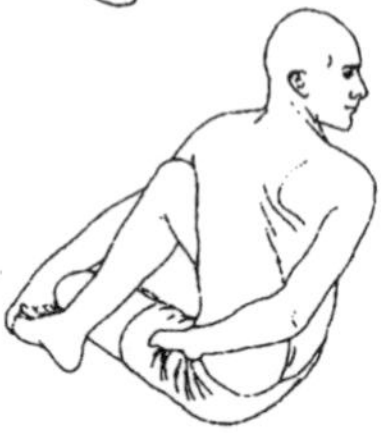	1 round (45 sec. each side)	p. 46
PAŠCIMATÂNÂSANA (Posterior Stretch Pose)	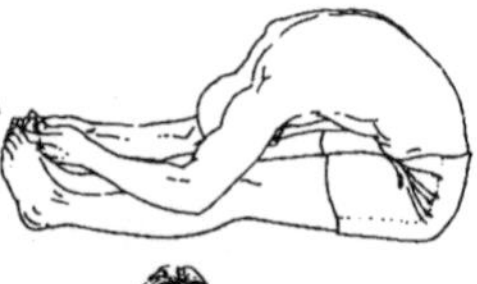	1 round (1 minute)	p. 49
SAṄKAṬÂSANA (Difficult Pose)	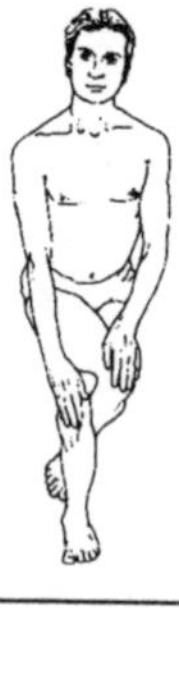	1 round (30 sec. each side)	p. 60

CAKRÂSANA (Side-Bending Pose)	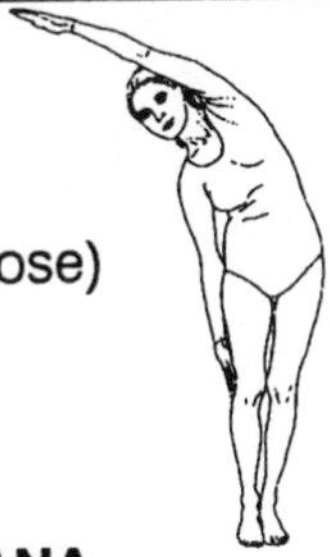	3 rounds (15 sec. each side)	p. 54
PÂDAHASTÂSANA (Hand-to-Foot Pose)	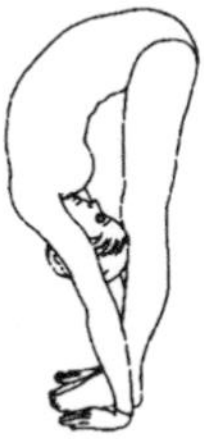	3 rounds (15 sec. each)	p. 63
BRAHMA MUDRÂ (Symbol of Brahmâ)	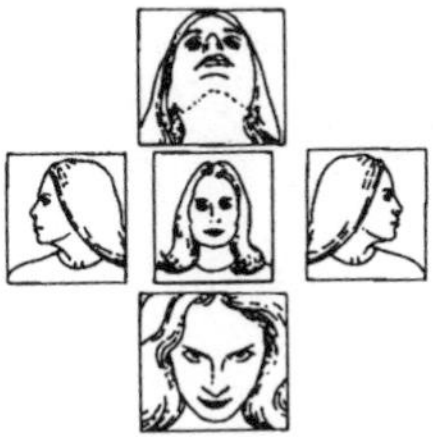	2 rounds (5 sec. each position)	p. 82
YOGA MUDRÂ (Symbol of Yoga)	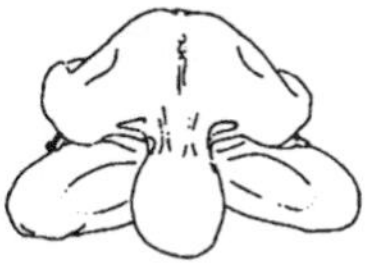	1 round (3 minutes)	p. 79
UJJÂYÎ (Breathing with Sound) first stage	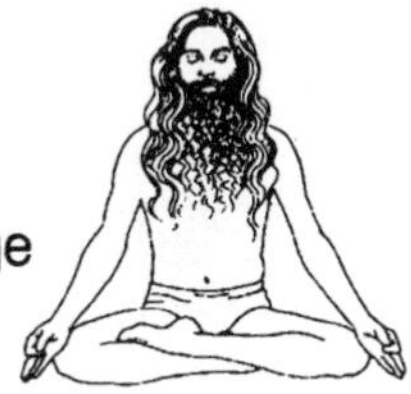	5 rounds	p. 85
UJJÂYÎ (Breathing with Sound) second stage	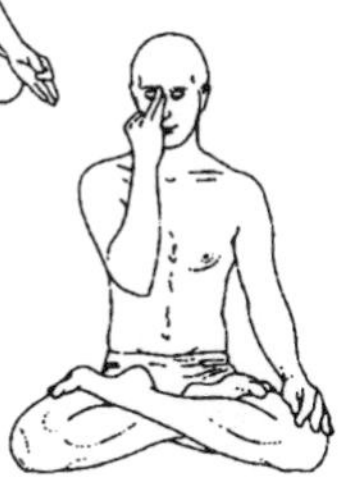	10 rounds	p. 88
ŠAVÂSANA (Corpse Pose)	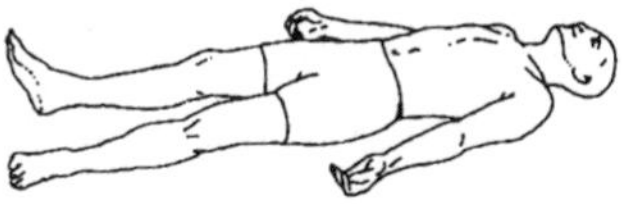	5 min.	p. 21

GLOSSARY

Abdominal Viscera, The interior organs in the great cavity of the abdomen.

Accomplished Pose, Siddhâsana

Adrenals, Supra-renal capsules; endocrine structures situated on top of the kidneys.

Âkâša Tattva, Ether element.

Âkṛṣya, Effortful lifting.

Anal Plexus, Pelvic plexus. Mûlâdhâra Cakra.

Ardha-Halâsana, Half-Plow Pose.

Ardha-Matsyendrâsana, Half-Spinal Twist Pose.

Ardha-Šalabhâsana, Half-Locust Pose.

Âsana, A Yogic pose. A seat. The third item of the Yogic curriculum.

Âsanas, A Yoga text by Swâmî Kuvalayânanda.

Âtman, The Self. The individual soul.

Auspicious Pose, Svastikâsana.

Baddha Padmâsana, Bound Lotus Pose.

Bandha, Lock. Certain neuro-muscular arrangements.

Bhujaṅgâsana, Cobra Pose.

Bound Lotus Pose, Baddha Padmâsana.

Bow Pose, Dhanurâsana.

Brahmâ, The Creator.

Brahma Mudrâ, Symbol of Brahmâ.

Brahman, The Supreme Being. The self existent spirit. The absolute.

Breathing with Sound, Ujjâyî Breathing.

Buddhist, A follower of the religion taught by Buddha.

Cakra, Padma. Lotus. Plexus. A circle or depression of the body. A nerve center of spiritual significance.

Cakrâsana, A wheel pose. In this text, Side-Bending Pose.

Cervical, That part of the vertebral column covering the neck.

Cobra Pose, Bhujaṅgâsana.

Corpse Pose, Šavâsana.

Crocodile Pose, Makarâsana.

Daṇḍâsana, Stick Pose.

Daršanopaniṣad, A sacred text of the Hindus.

Dhanurâsana, Bow Pose

Dhâraṇâ, Concentration. The fixing of the Citta (consciousness) on the impulses inside. The sixth item of the Yogic curriculum. Part of Internal Yoga.

Dhyâna, Meditation. Intensified Dhâraṇâ. The seventh item of the Yogic curriculum.

Difficult Pose, Saṅkaṭâsana.

Dorsal, That part of the spine which supports the back of the chest.

Earth Element, Pṛthvî Tattva.

Easy Pose, Sukhâsana.

Ether Element, Âkâša Tattva.

Gheraṇḍa Saṁhitâ, A text of Haṭha Yoga.

Gorakṣa Šatakam, A text of Haṭha Yoga.

Halâsana, Plow Pose.

Half-Locust Pose, Ardha-Šalabhâsana.

Half-Plow Pose, Ardha-Halâsana.

Half-Spinal Twist Pose, Ardha-Matsyendrâsana.

Hand-to-Foot Pose, Pâdahastâsana.

Haṭha-Pradîpikâ, A text of Haṭha Yoga.

Haṭha Yoga, That system of Yoga which starts with the purification of the body as the first step towards spiritual perfection.

Hero Pose, Vîrâsana.

Hypogastric Plexus, Svâdhiṣṭhâna Cakra.

Indra, The lord of gods. The god of rain.

Jñâna Mudrâ, Symbol of Knowledge.

Jugular Notch, The depression below the throat.

Kumbhaka, Breath retention in a particular manner. The phase of controlled suspension of breath.

Kuṇḍalinî, Serpent power or latent energy. The spiritual energy ordinarily sleeping in Mûlâdhâra.

Kuša, A sacred grass. (Poa Cynosuroides / Pampas Grass; a grass with long, pointed stalks.)

Latent Energy, Kuṇḍalinî.

Lac (Lakh), 100,000.

Lock, Bandha.

Locust Pose, Šalabhâsana.

Lord Kṛṣṇa, Viṣṇu in his eighth incarnation. Šrî Kṛṣṇa is the most celebrated hero of Indian mythology.

Lord Šiva, Name of the third god of the sacred Hindu trinity, who is entrusted with the work of involution as Brahmâ and Viṣṇu are with the evolution (creation) and preservation of the world.

Lotus Pose, Padmâsana.

Lumbo-Sacral, That part of the spine which supports from behind the abdomen and pelvis.

Maharṣi Patañjali, The celebrated author of the *Yoga Sûtras*. The first systematic exponent of Yoga philosophy.

Makarâsana, Crocodile Pose.

Maṇipur Cakra, Solar plexus. Epigastric plexus.

Mantra, Sacred prayer (addressed to any deity). Formula of worship.

Matsyendra Nâth, See Šrî Matsyendra Nâth.

Matsyendrâsana, The Spinal twist pose named after the ancient exponent of Haṭha Yoga, Šrî Matsyendra Nâth.

Meditation, Dhyâna.

Mṛtâsana, Šavâsana. Dead Man's Pose, or Corpse Pose.

Mudrâ, A symbol. A seal. One of the components of Haṭha Yoga.

Mûlâdhâra Cakra, Anal plexus. Pelvic plexus.

Muṇḍaka Upaniṣad, A sacred text of the Hindus.

Nâḍî, A nerve; a nostril.

Namaskâra Mudrâ, Indian way of Salutation.

Niyama, Any voluntary or self-imposed observance. The second item of the Yogic curriculum. According to Patañjali, the Niyamas are: cleanliness, contentment, austerities, self-study, and devotion or surrender to God.

Om, The sacred syllable.

Pâdahastâsana, Hand-To-Foot Pose.

Padmâsana, Lotus Pose.

Parathyroid, Accessory thyroid glands, four in number, situated on the dorsal aspect of the thyroid.

Paščimatânâsana, Posterior Stretch Pose.

Paščimottânâsana, Paščimatânâsana, Posterior Stretch Pose.

Patañjali, See Maharṣi Patañjali.

Pelvic Pose, Vajrâsana.

Pelvic Region, The lowermost part of the abdominal cavity between the hip bones.

Perineum, Region between the anus and genitals.

Pillar Pose, Stambhâsana.

Plexus, Cakra. Padma. Lotus. A network of nerves and blood vessels.

Plow Pose, Halâsana.

Posterior Stretch Pose, Paščimatânâsana.

Posture, Âsana. An attitude assumed by the body.

Prâṇâyâma, The fourth item of the Yogic curriculum. Yogic breath control. Kumbhaka.

Prâṇâyâma, A Yoga text by Swâmî Kuvalayânanda.

Prašvâsa, Normal exhalation.

Pratyâhâra, Sense withdrawal. The fifth item of the Yogic curriculum. Introversion of the mind.

Prone, Lying with the front or face downward.

Pṛthvî Tattva, Earth Element.

Pûraka, Breath inhalation in a particular manner. Controlled inspiratory phase.

Recaka, Breath exhalation in a particular manner. The phase of controlled expiration.

Sadâšiva, The deity of Višuddha Cakra.

Šalabhâsana, Locust Pose.

Samâdhi, The eighth and the last item of the Yogic curriculum. Perfect absorption of thought into an object of meditation. A state of harmony which is difficult to describe.

Saṅkaṭâsana, Difficult Pose.

Ṣaṭ-Cakra-Nirûpaṇa, A text of Tantra Yoga.

Šavâsana, Corpse Pose.

Serpent Power, Kuṇḍalinî.

Siddhâsana, Accomplished Pose.

Siddha-Siddhânta-Paddhati, A text of Haṭha Yoga.

Side-Bending Pose, Cakrâsana.

Šiva, Auspicious. See Lord Šiva.

Šiva-Saṁhitâ, A text of Haṭha Yoga.

Šivâsana, Seat of Lord Šiva.

Solar Plexus, Epigastric plexus. Maṇipur cakra.

Spinal Cord, A thin rope-like nervous structure attached to the brain and lodged in the spinal canal.

Spinal Nerve, Suṣumṇâ.

Spinal Twist Pose, Matsyendrâsana.

Šrî Matsyendra Nâth, The great ancient exponent of Haṭha Yoga.

Šrîmadbhagavadgîtâ, A sacred text of the Hindus.

Stambhâsana, Pillar Pose.

Stick Pose, Daṇḍâsana.

Sukhâsana, Easy Pose.

Šukra, The planet Venus. The name of the preceptor of Asuras. Life preserving spinal secretion.

Supine, Lying on the back or having the face upward.

Suṣumṇâ, The spinal nerve (cord).

Sûtra, An aphorism.

Švâsa, Normal inhalation.

Svâdhiṣṭhâna Cakra, Hypogastric Plexus.

Svastikâsana, Auspicious Pose.

Swâmî Kuvalayânanda, A pioneering exponent of the modern, scientific approach to classical Yoga, who founded Kaivalyadhâma Yoga Institute in India.

Symbol of Brahmâ, Brahma Mudrâ.

Symbol of Knowledge, Jñâna Mudrâ.

Tattva, Element.

Thyroid, An endocrine gland situated in the neck.

Tree Pose, Vṛkṣâsana.

Trišikhibrâhmṇopaniṣad, A sacred text of the Hindus.

Twist Pose, Vakrâsana.

Ugrâsana, Pašcimatânâsana, Posterior Stretch Pose.

Ujjâyî, Breathing with sound; breathing which leads to success. Effortful lifting of the breath from the navel.

Uttâna, Stretched.

Vâcasapati, One of the principal commentators of the *Yoga Sûtras*.

Vajrâsana, Pelvic Pose.

Vakrâsana, Twist Pose.

Varâhopaniṣad, A sacred text of the Hindus.

Varuṇa Bîja, Water seed.

Vedas, The holy scriptures of the Hindus.

Vertebra, Each of the thirty-three pieces which form the backbone.

Vîrâsana, Hero Pose.

Viscera, The interior organs in the great cavities of the body, especially in the abdomen.

Višuddha Cakra, Carotid plexus. One of the plexus situated at the throat.

Vṛkṣâsana, Tree Pose.

Vyâsa, A compiler. The name of a celebrated sage. The author of the great epic, *The Mahâbhârata*, and a commentator of the *Yoga Sûtras*. Several other works are also ascribed to him.

Vyomasaṁcâra, A feeling of floating in the sky.

Water Seed, Varuṇa Bîja

Yama, Restraint. The first item of the Yogic curriculum, which prescribes helpful rules for interpersonal relations. According to Patañjali, the Yamas are: non-harming; truthfulness; non-stealing; spiritual and disciplined life, Goal (Brahman)-orientedness, continence; non-possession.

Yoga, "A system of exercises, physical or mental, which may begin with the purification of the body and which culminate in a stage wherein the individual soul becomes merged into the Infinite." (Swâmî Kuvalayânanda)

A system of exercises which helps in regulating the behavior of consciousness in order to understand one's self.

Yogakuṇḍalinyupaniṣad, A sacred text of the Hindus.

Yoga Mudrâ, Symbol of Yoga.

Yoga Sûtras, Aphorisms on Yoga. Ancient and authoritative text on Yoga.

Yogic Therapy, A text of the science and art of healing by means of Yogic exercises.

Zazen, Sitting meditation.

References

ABBR.	TITLE	PARTICULARS
Â.	*Âsanas*	Kuvalayânanda, Swâmî. Kaivalyadhâma. Lonavla, India 1933.
D.U.	*Daršanopaniṣad*	Šastrî, A. Mahâdeva (Ed.). *The Yoga Upaniṣad-s*, The Adyar Library and Research Centre. Madras, India 1968.
Gh.S.	*Gheraṇḍa Saṁhitâ*	Vasu, S. C. (Trans.). Theosophical Publishing House. Adyar, Madras, India 1933.
		Digambarji, Swâmî and Gharote, M. L. (Ed.). Kaivalyadhâma S. M. Y. M. Samiti. Lonavla, India 1978.
GÎTÂ	*Šrîmadbhagavadgîtâ*	Swarupananda, Swâmî (Trans.). Advaita Ashrama. Calcutta, India 1976.
G.Š.	*Gorakṣa Šatakam*	Kuvalayânanda, Swâmî and Shukla, S. A. (Ed.). Kaivalyadhâma S. M. Y. M. Samiti. Lonavla, India 1958.

ABBR.	TITLE	PARTICULARS
H.P.	*Haṭha-Pradîpikâ*	Digambarji, Swâmî and Kokaje, R. G. (Ed.). Kaivalyadhâma S. M. Y. M. Samiti. Lonavla, India 1970.
M.U.	*Muṇḍaka Upaniṣad*	Gambhîrânanda, Swâmî (Ed.). *Eight Upaniṣads*, Volume 2. Advaita Ashrama. Calcutta, India 1966.
P.	*Prâṇâyâma*	Kuvalayânanda, Swâmî. Kaivalyadhâma. Lonavla, India 1931.
P.Y.S.	*Patañjali's Yoga Sûtras*	Prasâda, Râma (Trans.). Sudhindranath Vasu, Pâṇini Office, Bhuvaneśwarî Âsrama, Bahadurganj, Allahabad, India 1924.
		Woods, J. H. (Trans.). *The Yoga-System of Patañjali,* Motilal Banarsidass. Delhi, India 1966.
		Pâtañjala Yoga Darśanam, Chaukhamba Sanskrit Series. Benaras, India 1934.
		Digambarji, Swâmî. *Transliteration and Easy Rendering of Patañjali's Yoga Sutras,* SKY, Number 14. Kaivalyadhâma. Lonavla, India 1987.

ABBR.	TITLE	PARTICULARS
Ṣ.C.N.	*Ṣaṭ-Cakra-Nirûpaṇa*	Woodroffe, Sir J. (Trans.). *The Serpent Power*. Ganesh & Co.. Madras, India 1973.
S.S.P.	*Siddha-Siddhânta-Paddhati*	Šrî Gorakṣanâtha. Šrî Pûrṇa Nâthaji, Šrî Yogâšrama Sanskrit College. Bohar, India 1939.
		Mallik, K. *Siddha-Siddhânta-Paddhati and Other Works of Nath Yogis,* Poona Oriental Book House. Poona, India 1954.
Š.S.	*Šiva-Saṁhitâ*	Vidyârṇava, Š. C. (Trans.). Lalit Mohan Basu, Pâṇini Office, Sukumari Ashram, Allahabad, India 1942.
T.Š.B.	*Trišikhibrâhmṇopaniṣad*	Šastrî, A. Mahâdeva (Ed.). *The Yoga Upaniṣad-s*, The Adyar Library and Research Centre. Madras, India 1968.
V.U.	*Varâhopaniṣad*	Šastrî, A. Mahâdeva (Ed.). *The Yoga Upaniṣad-s*, The Adyar Library and Research Centre. Madras, India 1968.
Y.K.U.	*Yogakuṇḍalinyupaniṣad*	Šastrî, A. Mahâdeva (Ed.). *The Yoga Upaniṣad-s*, The Adyar Library and Research Centre. Madras, India 1968.

Y.T. *Yogic Therapy* Kuvalayânanda, Swâmî and Vinekar, S. L. Kaivalyadhâma S. M. Y. M. Samiti, Lonavla, India 1963.

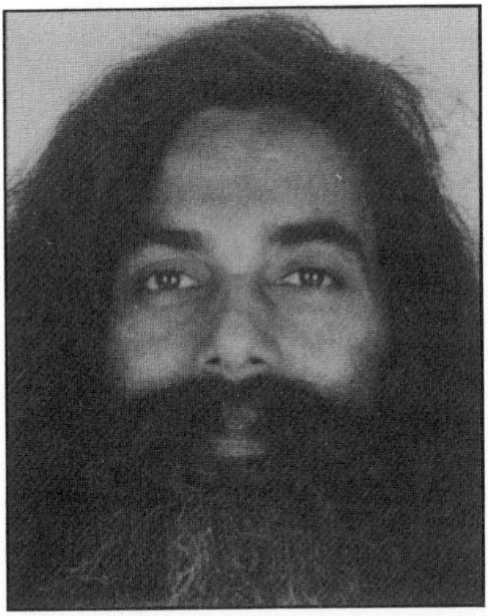

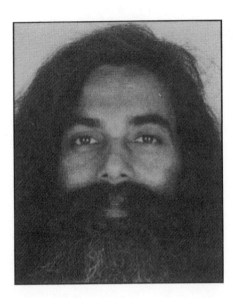

Dr. Vijayendra Pratap is the founder/director of the Swami Kuvalayananda Yoga (SKY) Foundation and the Yoga Research Society. He earned his Ph.D. from the Department of Applied Psychology, University of Bombay. He served at India's Kaivalyadhama Yoga Institute as Lecturer of Yoga and Mental Health, Assistant Director of Scientific Research, and Managing Editor of YOGA MIMAMSA.

Dr. Pratap has conducted Yoga programs for institutions worldwide, including the following: Institute of Religious Psychology, Tokyo; Association for Humanistic Psychology, Eastern Regional Conferences, Philadelphia and Atlantic City; Esalen, Big Sur, California; Tulsa Psychiatric Center, Tulsa; University of New Mexico School of Medicine; Spring Yoga Festival, Ananda Ashram, New York; Association for Transpersonal Psychology Conference, Stanford University; Jefferson University, Philadelphia; Instituto Psicosomatica E Yoga, Torino, Italy; the Pan American Commission for Yoga, Sao Paulo, Brazil; and the Yoga for Peace International Conference, Jerusalem, Israel.

Dr. Pratap has made presentations at various conferences, such as: the World Conference of Scientific Yoga, New Delhi; the XXth International Congress of Psychology, Tokyo; the Biofeedback Research Society Conference, Colorado; the International Yoga and Meditation Congresses, Chicago; the Third World Congress of Yoga, Sao Paulo; and the Yoga Research Society Conferences, Philadelphia.